Easy and Tasty Recipes with Pictures

ARTHRITIS
Action Guide
& Cookbook

Libby Nau

Copyright © 2023 by Sunny Spot Publishing, Florida

All rights reserved. No part of this publication may be reproduced, stored in or introduced into a retrieval system, or transmitted, in any form, or by any means (electronic, mechanical, photocopying, recording, or otherwise) without the prior written permission of the copyright owner of this book.

The author of this book does not dispense medical advice or prescribe the use of any technique as a form of treatment for physical, emotional, or medical problems without the advice of a physician, either directly or indirectly. The intent of the author is only to offer information of a general nature to help you in your quest for knowledge. In the event you use any of the information in this book for yourself, the author and the publisher assume no responsibility for your actions.

This book is not intended as a substitute for the medical advice of physicians. The reader should regularly consult a physician in health matters, particularly about any symptoms that may require diagnosis or medical attention. This book is solely for educational purposes and does not constitute medical advice. Please consult a medical or health professional before you begin any exercise, nutrition, or supplementation program or if you have questions about your health.

Dedication

This book is for my family –

Your love, support, and encouragement make everything possible. We do not know what we are capable of until we try, so reach for your dreams. Find the lesson in every outcome, and be grateful for the experience. Above all, be kind to yourself and others, and do all things with love.

Acknowledgments

The recipes in this cookbook were created by Philippa Grylls, a food scientist with a Master's degree in Food Science. Philippa is passionate about science, health, and nutrition, and she specializes in recipe development for specific dietary requirements. An avid researcher, she keeps up-to-date with the latest scientific research. Philippa's expertise, dedication, and attention to detail were invaluable to this project.

CONTENTS

CONTENTS

Dedication	i
Acknowledgments	ii
Introduction	1
This book is divided into four parts	3

PART 1

My Arthritis Story	5
What I've Done To Manage Symptoms	10

PART 2

Arthritis: A Quick Overview	16
What Causes It?	17
Common Types of Arthritis	18
A Proper Diagnosis	19
What Can You Do About It?	21

PART 3

Benefits of Anti-Inflammatory Foods	24
Anti-inflammatory Foods – Eat These!	27
Inflammatory Foods – Avoid These!	30
References	32

PART 4

Arthritis Cookbook	**34**
The Recipes	**35**
Master Shopping List	**36**
Oatmeal Berry Bowl with Nuts and Orange Slices	**39**
Triple Yum Yogurt with Muesli, Nuts, and Berries	**41**
Oat and Banana Pancakes	**43**
Breakfast Burrito	**47**
Tuna Salad with Leafy Green & Fresh Vegetables	**51**
Grain and Veggie "Buddha" Bowl	**53**
Penne Pasta with Tomato & Grilled Green Vegetables	**57**
Pitas with Falafels and Hummus	**61**

Butternut Squash Soup	**63**
Baked Salmon with Fresh & Savory Green Vegetables	**67**
Baked Chicken with Red Peppers and Sweet Potato	**71**
Creamy Avocado Pasta with Green Beans and Cabbage	**75**
Vegetable Stir-Fry – Chicken Stir-Fry	**79**
Chocolate Chia Pudding with Blueberries	**83**
Nut Butter Banana Smoothie	**85**
About the Author	**87**
Customer reviews	**88**

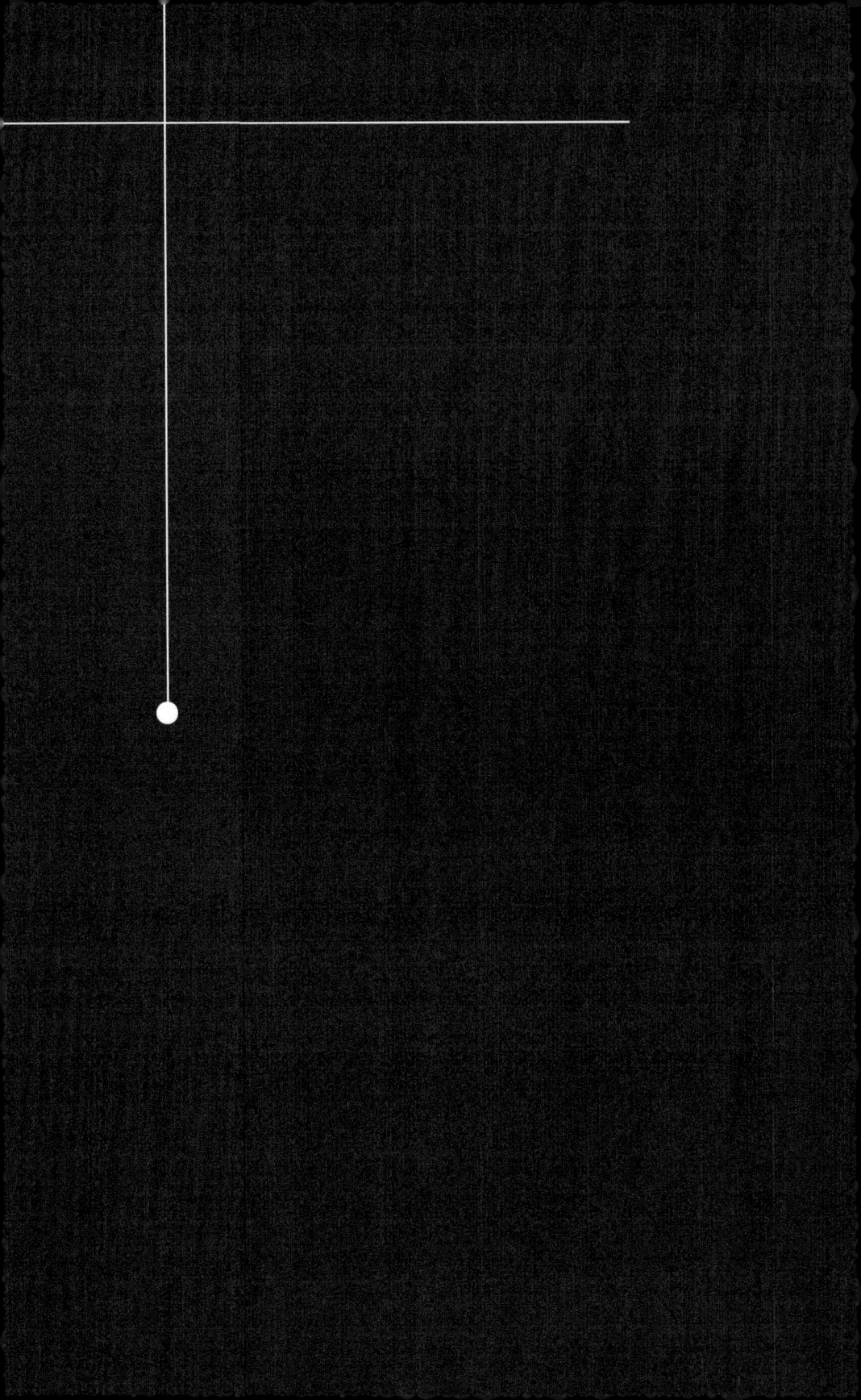

Introduction

When I was in my early 20s, my husband's Aunt Helen liked to share an often-told joke. Every now and then, she'd casually mention that she'd had a visit from "Arthur."

"Arthur? Arthur, who?" we'd ask.

"Arthur Ritis," she'd say with a pained smile, rubbing her swollen hands. Oh, right. She meant ARTHRITIS. Then we'd sympathize and laugh along with her. She was such a good sport and always willing to lend a helping hand, even if she was hurting.

Like many elderly people I know, she took her aches and pains in stride, an inevitable sign of aging. People who use their hands a lot, for work or recreation, usually minimize their pain and say, "No use in complaining. It won't do any good." Ha ha ha!

Now that I'm in my 50s, I'm starting to get visits from "Arthur," and it's not so funny. I wish he'd stay away because the pain he brings is nothing to laugh about.

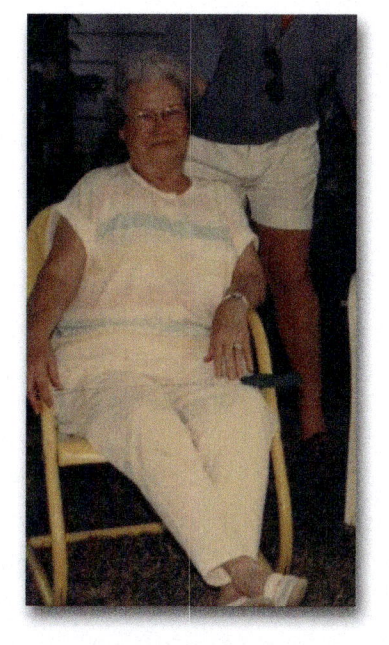

Aunt Helen and her hard-working hands

With that in mind, I wrote the *Arthritis Action Guide & Cookbook: Easy and Tasty Recipes with Pictures*. Over the last few years,

I've learned a lot about arthritis and what I can do to relieve my symptoms. I'm not an expert, but I do have arthritis and it's taught me some lessons that I want to share. Although there is no cure for arthritis, you can take action to make it more manageable. I hope you can benefit from my experience and reduce your arthritis pain.

Good luck and best wishes for your better health!

Libby

This book is divided into four parts

Part 1

My Arthritis Story. How arthritis has affected me and what I've done to manage it.

Part 2

Arthritis: A Quick Overview. What it is, what causes it, common types, the importance of getting a proper diagnosis, and what you can do about it.

Part 3

Benefits of Anti-inflammatory Foods. Discover which foods help reduce inflammation and ease painful arthritis symptoms. Includes lists of foods to eat and avoid.

Part 4

An Arthritis Cookbook: Easy and Tasty Recipes With Pictures. Features 15 original anti-inflammatory recipes for breakfast, lunch, dinner, and dessert. Each recipe is accompanied by a full-color picture, nutrition facts, and simple step-by-step directions. A master shopping list shows all the ingredients needed.

PART 1

My Arthritis Story

Just a few years ago, I had a sign-painting business that I loved. To make my custom signs, I used a jigsaw to cut scrap wood, then I'd smooth the surface with a palm sander. Once the wood was prepped, I painted on the lettering and then added a protective coat of polyurethane. To finish, I drilled screws to the back and attached heavy-gauge wire to make a hanger. The work was enjoyable, and I didn't mind the repetitive tasks.

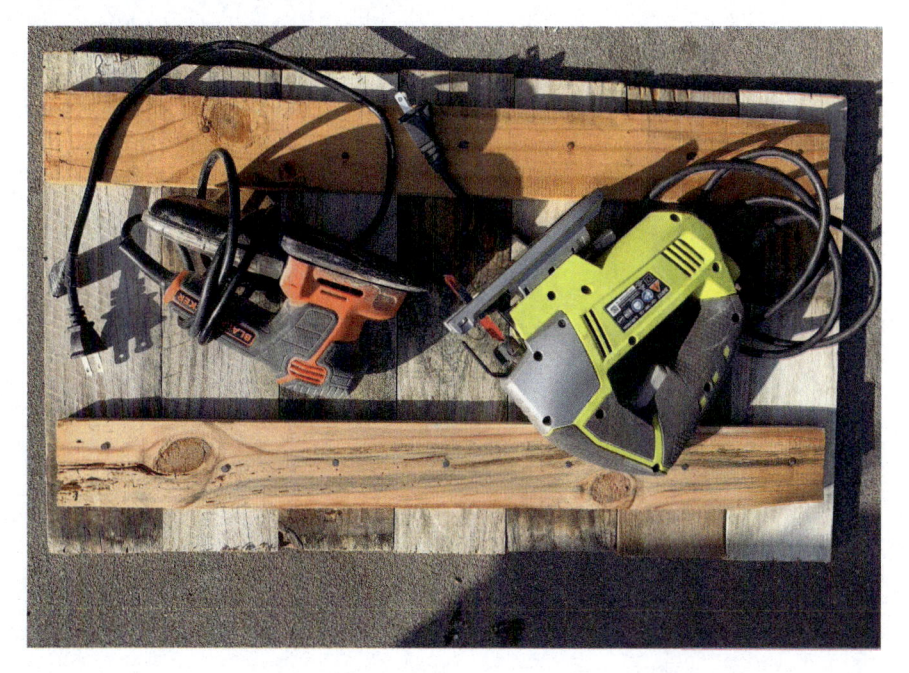

My two favorite power tools: a jigsaw and a palm sander

At the end of a busy day of cutting wood, my hands were numb from the constant vibration of the power tools. By the next day, however, my hands had recovered and were ready to do the less strenuous work of painting. By alternating cutting days and painting days, I was able to manage my discomfort.

At the same time, I was also teaching a fine art acrylic painting class for beginners at the local craft store. To demonstrate specific painting techniques, I needed my fingers to be flexible and strong enough to show how to hold a paintbrush to make it do what you want. The weekly classes were fun and didn't feel like work, much like my sign painting.

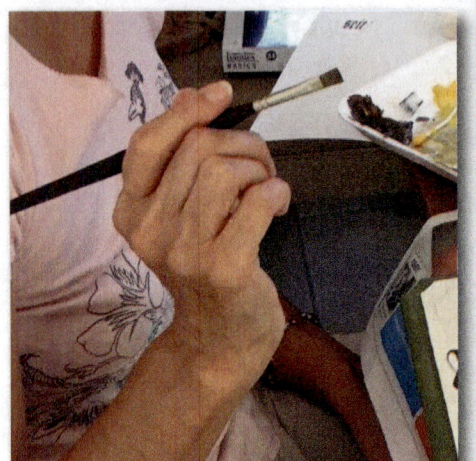

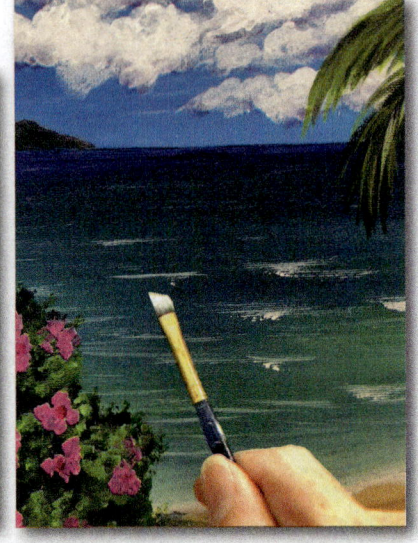

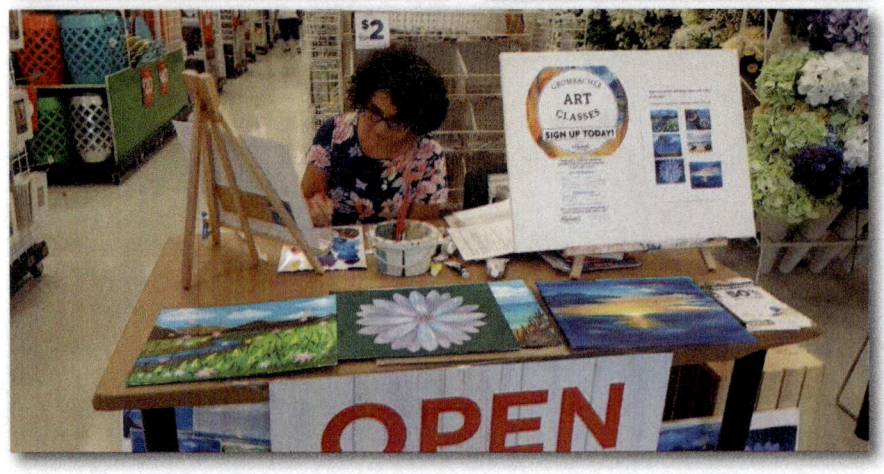

Teaching painting classes for beginners – a fun and relaxing activity

6

Examples of my signs – lots of cutting and sanding wood before painting

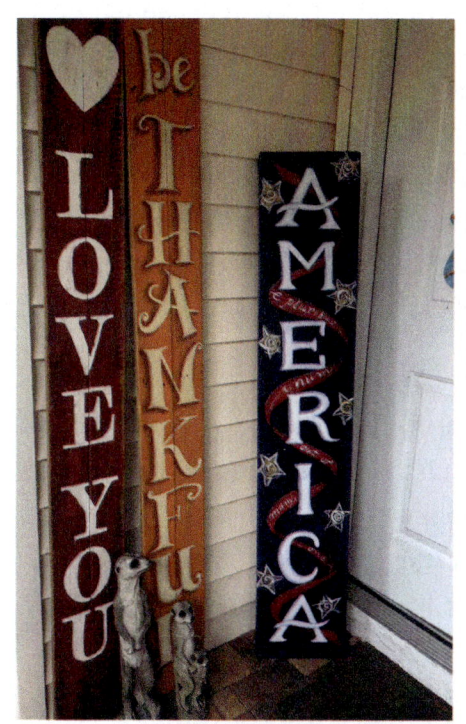

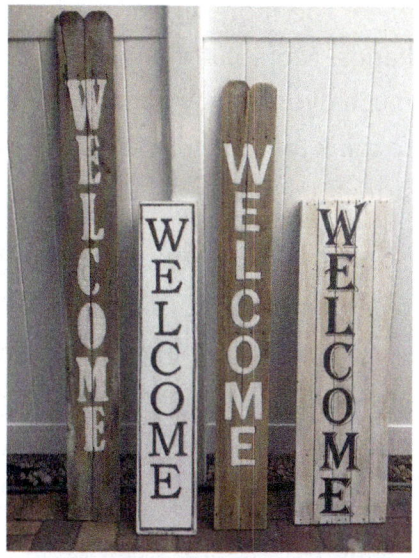

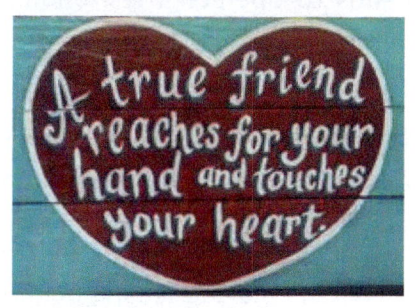

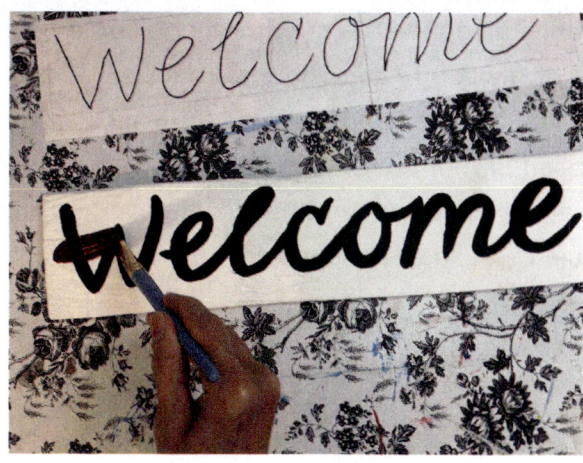

Eventually, as the saying goes, "All good things must come to an end." The more signs I made, the more stress I was putting on my hands. More cutting meant more time needed to recover. With so much overuse, my hands were often sore and weak. When I started to think twice before starting a new project, I realized I needed to do something.

Have you overused your hands like I did, perhaps with another type of repetitive activity? Maybe you play a musical instrument, sew, or work in the garden. Have you started to notice more aches and pains? Even pleasurable activities if overdone can cause pain or discomfort.

In the modern era, it's almost impossible to avoid using your hands to operate a cell phone or type on a computer keyboard. Other everyday activities that require hands include preparing food for cooking, gripping a steering wheel while driving, or using a can opener. All this repetitive activity can begin to add up and affect your hands. It's easy to take for granted having strong, flexible hands and fingers until you start to have a problem.

When I started feeling pain in my hands and wrist that wouldn't go away, I made an appointment with my doctor. After a thorough examination of my stiff fingers, bumpy knuckles, and tender wrist, she zeroed in on my right hand basal joint, the area around the wrist and the webbed part of the thumb. It wasn't hard to figure out that I had overused my hands. All that time spent overworking my hands had consequences; I had developed arthritis.

My type of arthritis, known as osteoarthritis, is likely a result of overuse and often worsens with age.

Despite the prognosis, my doctor was encouraging and recommended the following treatment:

1. Wear a hand and wrist brace
2. Use an over-the-counter pain reliever
3. Practice gentle exercises
4. Eat anti-inflammatory foods

WHAT I'VE DONE TO MANAGE SYMPTOMS

To prevent my arthritis from getting worse, I decided to cut back on the main source of my problem: using power tools that put undue stress on my hands. I stopped cutting wood for my signs and began to phase out my sign painting business. I focused more on my painting classes since they required much less strenuous and repetitive hand motions.

Wear Hand and Wrist Braces

Following my doctor's advice, I started wearing a hand and wrist brace. There are many variations available, all designed to protect sore hands, reduce pain, and prevent further damage. These devices are helpful in immobilizing your hands so they can rest, but they are often uncomfortable and inconvenient to wear for long periods. Here are some that I've tried:

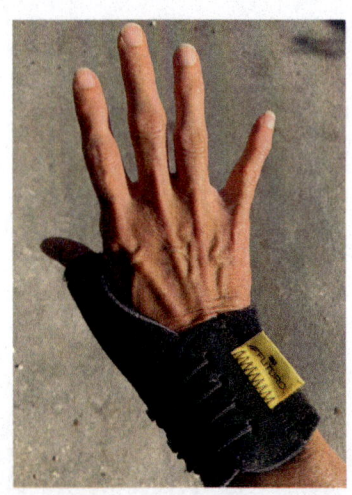

Futuro wrist support: Keeps thumb protected and easy to wear; not much support but keeps area warm

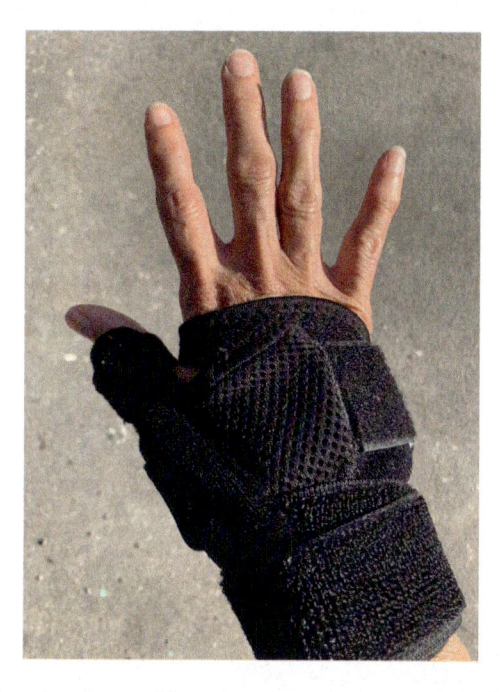

Dr. Arthritis fitted wrist and hand support brace: Much thicker support keeps wrist and thumb stable but hard to keep on for long periods

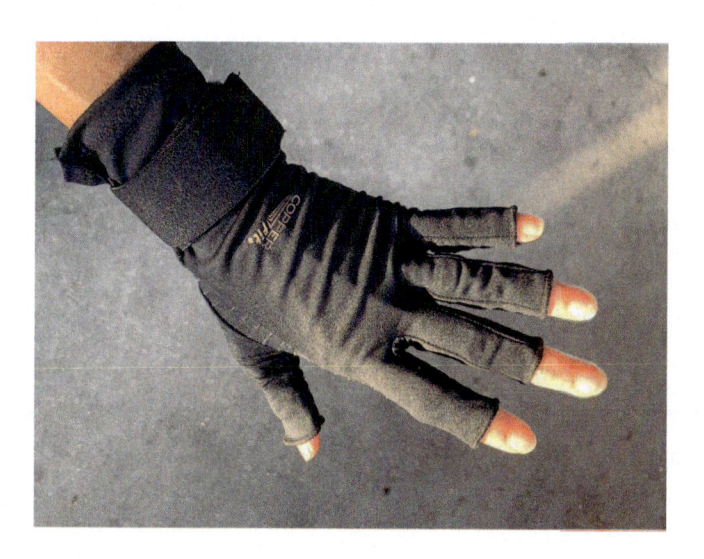

Copperfit compression gloves: Very soft and comfortable, keeps hands warm but not much relief for pain

Use an Over-the-Counter Pain Reliever

My doctor suggested using an over-the-counter pain reliever (Voltaren) to relieve pain, up to 4 times a day. This has provided temporary relief when I use it; however, it is a strong medication, and precautions must be taken. You must follow directions exactly for it to be effective.

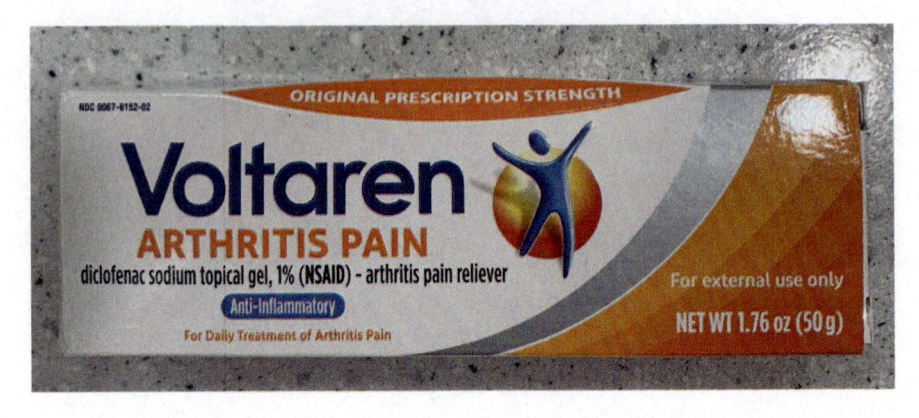

Voltaren, a popular over-the-counter pain relief aid for arthritis

Practice Gentle Exercise

To find gentle exercises, I searched online for "arthritis exercises hands" and found several links to helpful videos showing easy-to-do exercises. I tried several and settled on a few that I liked. Now I use hand and finger exercises regularly to keep my finger joints strong and flexible. For me, the best movements gently stretch and flex the finger joints. You can do them any time your hands feel stiff, and they will help improve your range of motion and strength.

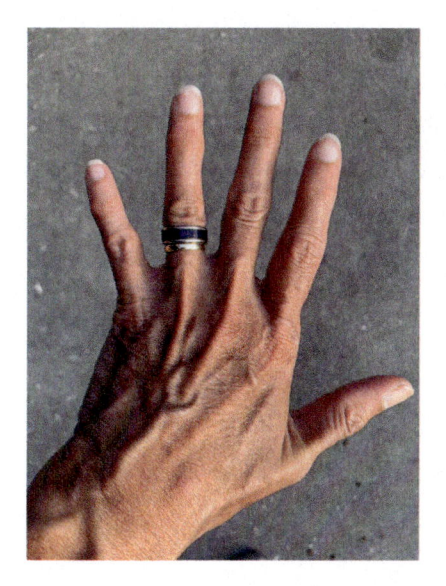

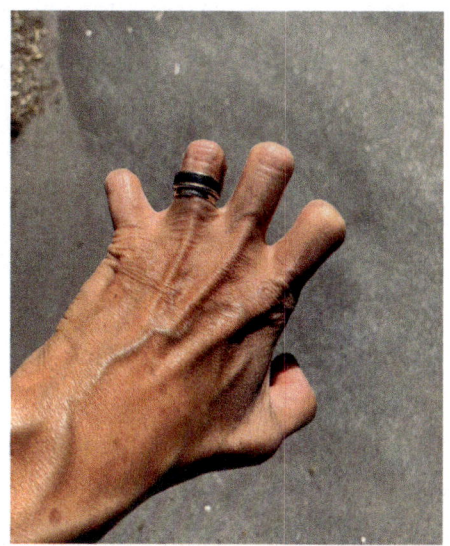

Hand exercises to relieve joint pain

My favorite exercise is what I call "Stretch and Scrunch." To do this, extend the fingers on each hand with a full stretch. Then retract the fingers into a claw, bending at the joints. Repeat several times, whenever your fingers feel stiff.

Eat Anti-Inflammatory Foods

My doctor also recommended trying an anti-inflammatory diet. These diets are popular and can help relieve arthritis symptoms.

If you're like me, you're interested in finding ways to live pain-free, within reason. The "cure" shouldn't taste horrible, make you feel ill, or cause even more discomfort than the condition you want to treat. I'm willing to try (almost) anything to improve my quality of life, but it has to be doable, affordable, and convenient enough for me to stick with it. Recipes, even healthy anti-inflammatory ones, should be tasty enough that you'd want to eat them.

After reviewing several anti-inflammatory diets, I asked a food scientist to develop a small collection of recipes, designed for a beginner. To be effective, the recipes had to be easy to make, use ingredients that were readily available at local grocery stores, and be tasty enough that you'd want to make them again.

I tested all the recipes to make sure that they truly are easy and tasty. (They are!) I found that when I eat better, I feel better. I encourage you to try a recipe or two and assess how you feel. You might be surprised at how easy it is to add anti-inflammatory foods to your diet. These recipes are featured in Part 4, the cookbook portion of this book.

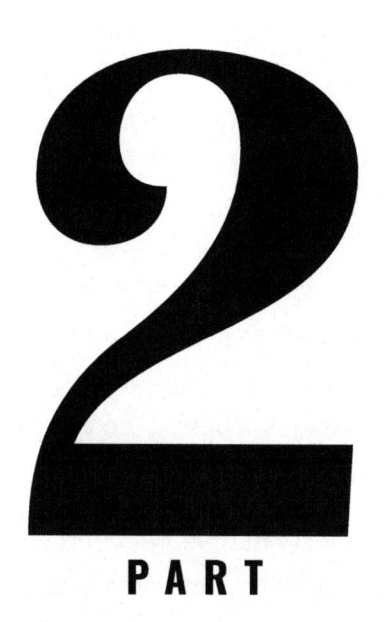

PART 2

Arthritis: A Quick Overview

Are your wrists sore when you wake up in the morning? Do your ankles hurt after a stroll? Maybe your knee joints crack when you get up from a chair or your fingers hurt when you try to open a jar. If you experience discomfort, stiffness, and a reduced range of movement in your joints, you might have arthritis.

What Is It?

Arthritis literally means "joint inflammation." It is not a single illness or disease but rather a catch-all phrase encompassing more than 100 conditions that damage the body's joints, tissues around the joints, and other connective tissues. There is no cure for arthritis, but you can take steps to manage the symptoms.

Arthritis generally affects people between the ages of 20 and 50, but it can affect all ages, even infants. The average age of onset is 47, and about three out of every five people with arthritis are under 65.

Symptoms range from moderate to severe and may appear and disappear over time. Some conditions may remain stable for years, then might increase and worsen with time.

In its early stages, arthritis makes daily tasks challenging. Joint stiffness makes it difficult to grip, hold, bend, reach, and lift. In its advanced stages, arthritis is excruciatingly painful and incapacitating.

What Causes It?

The exact science of what causes arthritis is still being researched. For most forms of arthritis, the causes are unknown. Injury, overuse of joints, and mechanical issues with joints (such as skeletal abnormalities or worn out joint muscles) can lead to arthritis. Heredity, stress, drugs, food allergies, and viruses have been linked to some forms of arthritis, as have diet, poor circulation, and lack of movement.

Although arthritis affects different sections of the body, they all have one thing in common: inflammation.

Common Types of Arthritis

The most common form of arthritis is osteoarthritis (OA). Other forms include rheumatoid arthritis, gout, and lupus.

Osteoarthritis (OA) and rheumatoid arthritis (RA) both have similar symptoms but different causes. OA occurs when joints are overused and misused, such as when the cartilage that protects the joint breaks down, and bones rub together. This generally happens in the knees, but can also occur in the hips, spine, and hands. Often it is only in the later stages that a person feels pain, after quite a bit of cartilage is already lost.

Rheumatoid arthritis occurs when the body's immune system attacks joint tissue. This condition most often starts in the hands, wrists, and feet and then advances to the shoulders, elbows, and hips. Symptoms include pain, stiffness, fatigue, weakness, slight fever, and inflamed tissue.

A Proper Diagnosis

If you suspect you have arthritis, early detection and treatment are important. Healthcare providers can help determine if your symptoms are arthritis or something else. If left untreated, arthritis can worsen and cause damage that cannot be undone or reversed.

A good place to start is by making an appointment with your healthcare provider to discuss your symptoms. With a proper diagnosis, you can find out more about your condition and learn about treatment options.

To prepare for your visit, think of questions ahead of time and be ready to take notes. Some questions to ask may include these:

- Do I have arthritis? If not, what is wrong and what do I do next? If so, which type is it? And what can I expect in the short- and long-term?
- What pain relief treatments are available? Which have side effects and what are they?
- What self-care solutions do you advise?
- Are there any limitations I should know about; for example, special dietary issues, special activities to avoid, any over-the-counter medication to consider, etc.?
- What recommendations do you have in the areas of diet and exercise?

Along with your questions, write down a list of your symptoms so your doctor can help better understand your situation. Make sure to note the following:

- Where you feel pain (same joint, both limbs?)
- When you feel pain (with certain activities, in the morning, when it rains, etc.)
- How long you have had the pain
- If the pain increases or decreases, comes and goes, etc.
- Type and intensity level of pain (stabbing, dull, cramping, stiffness; low, mild, or high)
- Impact and limitations (can't bend over too far without pain, can't get out of a car, etc.)
- Family history of arthritis
- Any over-the-counter or prescription medications or other treatments you currently take or use
- Any special diet or exercise program you may be following

What Can You Do About It?

If you are diagnosed with arthritis, take steps to avoid or slow the onset of symptoms.

Even if you have a hereditary susceptibility to arthritis, you can help postpone or minimize the advancement of the disease by making some lifestyle changes. These changes will help you maintain your bone health, decrease inflammation, and avoid the further development of arthritis and other related diseases.

Here are some lifestyle changes you can make right now:

Minimize Repeated Tasks

Manual labor, computer work, and certain kinds of sports and hobbies, if done repeatedly, can put excess strain on certain joints and weaken bone and joint tissue over time. Are there any repeated movements you make that might be causing you pain or damage? If so, cut back or find alternatives. Take short breaks throughout the day to allow your joints to relax.

If you play sports or engage in physical activities, take time to relax periodically and practice gentle exercise to reduce the risk of injury. Moderate, regular exercise can help reduce the progression of arthritis by strengthening the muscles around a joint to provide overall support.

Stop Smoking

If you need additional motivation to kick the habit (in addition to preventing lung disease and emphysema), consider this: smoking might worsen arthritis. Look into treatments that can help you stop smoking, especially if past attempts were unsuccessful. Cigarette smoking raises your chances of getting rheumatoid arthritis and may cause other medical issues.

Keep an Ideal Weight

Keeping an ideal weight through diet and exercise will lessen your risk of developing arthritis, as well as cardiovascular disease, obesity, and diabetes. Obesity directly impacts how much stress you put on your joints, which can cause inflammation. Knee and hip joints, where extra weight can cause progressive damage to your joints, are especially vulnerable to inflammation.

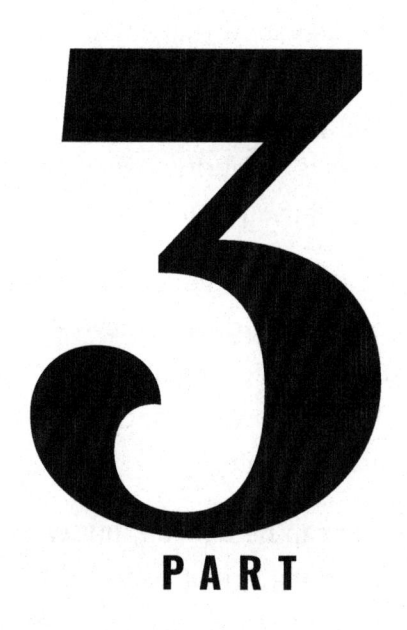

PART 3

Benefits of Anti-Inflammatory Foods

It is far better to treat an inflammatory condition early on than wait until it gets worse. Studies show that eating the right foods can help you reduce inflammation, the leading cause of pain and discomfort in the body. Controlling your food intake and restricting or reducing some problematic foods is a priority if you want to relieve the pain and stiffness of arthritis caused by inflammation.

While there's a great deal of debate in the medical world about the effect of diet on arthritis, doctors have known for a long time that diet affects gout, a specific type of arthritic condition. It's worth noting that several studies show that anti-inflammatory foods can be beneficial and ease arthritis pain.

Adopting a new diet can be difficult, but with the right mindset, you can make simple changes that can lead to big results in your overall health. I feel better when I eat food that helps me function at my best. From personal experience, I know that certain foods may taste delicious but they can make my body feel achy and tired.

Here are some steps you can take to start your anti-inflammatory lifestyle:

1. Learn to cook easy and tasty meals that incorporate anti-inflammatory foods.

2. Eat a variety of fruits, vegetables, lean proteins, dairy, nuts, cereals, and whole grains.
3. Avoid processed foods such as sweets, fried food, and pre-packaged dinners
4. Drink plenty of water.
5. Consider keeping a food diary or journal. Track your food consumption and note any symptoms you experience. This habit will help you better understand which foods may be causing problems. You may want to discuss your findings with your doctor.

Keep in mind that our bodies each process food in different ways. For instance, some foods can reduce pain for one person but may trigger more pain in another.

When trying new foods, use trial and error to determine which foods are best to incorporate into your diet. Only you know how your body reacts to a particular food. For example, there is conflicting information about the benefits of tomatoes and peppers, also known as "nightshade" vegetables, yet they are often on lists of foods recommended for an anti-inflammatory diet.

The Arthritis Foundation, a nonprofit organization that addresses the needs of people living with arthritis in the United States, recommends nightshades. The best strategy is to evaluate how you feel after eating certain foods and decide whether to continue eating them based on your experience.

It's important to note that the symptoms of arthritis, especially inflammatory arthritis, might vary for no apparent cause. Any improvement in your symptoms may not be caused by what you eat or changes you make to your diet. Therefore, it's better to make small changes, take notes, and review the results. Over time, you will get a better idea of how your diet is affecting your condition.

And, since everyone's nutritional demands vary, it's a good idea to consult with a doctor before starting an anti-inflammatory diet and lifestyle. For example, you shouldn't eliminate entire food categories from your diet, such as all dairy products, without trusted advice, since you may already be deficient in certain vitamins and minerals, and an arbitrary change might be detrimental to your overall health.

Finally, try to remember that an anti-inflammatory diet is not just about weight loss. That frozen "lean" meal may help you lose weight, but it isn't anti-inflammatory. The goal should be to eat foods that help you reduce inflammation so you can ease pain, build stamina, and lessen the pain of arthritis.

It's never too late to start a healthy lifestyle, and you can start right now in your kitchen! The following section lists recommended foods to eat and avoid.

Anti-inflammatory Foods – Eat These!

Red chili pepper

Also known as cayenne pepper, red chili pepper flakes or powder can help relieve joint pain associated with most types of arthritis.

Fish

Salmon, mackerel, sardines, and trout are rich in omega-3 fatty acids, which have been found to have significant anti-inflammatory benefits. Several studies have demonstrated that omega-3 fatty acid supplements can help reduce the degree of pain and morning stiffness of problematic joints.

The Arthritis Foundation suggests eating 3-6 ounces of fish two to four times each week to benefit from its anti-inflammatory qualities.

Garlic

Garlic is nutritious and flavorful and contains anti-inflammatory compounds that may even help prevent cartilage damage from arthritis.

Ginger

Ginger is widely used to fight inflammation. Available as a spice, it can be sprinkled on cooked vegetables and other foods. Fresh ginger is easy to peel and cook and can be kept frozen for months.

Oils

Extra virgin olive oil includes a high concentration of oleocanthal, which has anti-inflammatory characteristics similar to nonsteroidal anti-inflammatory medications (NSAIDs).

Broccoli

Cruciferous vegetables, such as broccoli, are among the healthiest foods and may help decrease inflammation. They contain glucosinolates, which have anti-inflammatory properties.

Dark Leafy Greens

Dark leafy greens, such as spinach, kale, chard, and collard greens, are high in vitamin D, anti-stress phytochemicals, and antioxidants. Vitamin D, which is required for calcium absorption, can stimulate the immune system, assisting the body in fighting illness.

Pineapple

Pineapple contains an enzyme called bromelain, which helps prevent inflammation in both osteoarthritis and rheumatoid arthritis. It's best to consume pineapple fresh instead of canned or frozen.

Walnuts

Walnuts are high in nutrients and contain chemicals that may help decrease inflammation linked with joint disorders. Walnuts are also abundant in alpha-linolenic acid, an omega-3 fatty acid found in plant diets. Omega-3 fatty acids have been found to decrease inflammation.

Dairy

Calcium and vitamin D are abundant in milk, yogurt, and cheese. These nutrients strengthen bones, which may alleviate the painful symptoms of arthritis. Dairy also includes proteins that can aid in muscle development.

Berries

Berries include a high concentration of antioxidants, vitamins, and minerals, which may account for their particular capacity to reduce inflammation. Strawberries, blackberries, and blueberries can satisfy cravings for sweets while providing arthritis-fighting nutrients.

Grapes

Grapes are a substantial source of antioxidants, which have anti-inflammatory qualities. Nutrient-dense, grapes also contain numerous substances proven to be effective in treating arthritis, such as resveratrol, an antioxidant in grape skin.

Green Tea

Green tea has an abundance of polyphenols, antioxidants that may be able to reduce inflammation and delay the deterioration of cartilage.

Inflammatory Foods – Avoid These!

Added Sugars

Sugar consumption causes inflammation in the body. It takes just 40 grams, or approximately the amount in one can of soda, to cause inflammation. Eliminating soft drinks, candies, and pastries may help decrease discomfort.

High-Fat Foods

Not all fats are created equal. To help protect your heart and preserve other organ functions, you need certain beneficial fats, such as those found in avocados, olive oil, and nuts. Trans fats, on the other hand, such as those found in processed meals, fried foods, fast foods, and doughnuts, can promote inflammation.

Carbohydrates

Carbs from meals are converted to energy by your body. That's why some athletes "carb load" before a race. But, refined carbs in white bread, white rice, and potato chips are a kind of carbohydrate that, if not transformed into energy to help you run a race, can remain in your system and lead to inflammation, excess weight, and other chronic conditions.

Tobacco and Alcoholic Beverages

These substances are hazardous to your general health and are known to cause inflammation, which may contribute to certain forms of arthritis. Smoking raises your chances of developing rheumatoid arthritis, and drinking has been related to gout and arthritis.

Gluten

Even if you don't have celiac disease (a disorder that destroys your small intestine), you should avoid gluten because it is known to cause joint inflammation. Choose gluten-free or whole wheat options.

Processed Food

Packaged food is easy to prepare and simplifies today's hectic lifestyle, but it can also exacerbate your arthritis symptoms. Manufacturers add monosodium glutamate (MSG), aspartame, and salt to preserve and improve food flavor. However, these chemicals have been related to increased inflammation. Avoiding processed meals, diet drinks, and other convenience items will also help reduce inflammation.

References

"Fast Facts About Arthritis." https://www.cdc.gov/arthritis/basics/arthritis-fast-facts.html. CDC. (2023).

"About Arthritis and RA." https://globalranetwork.org/project/disease-info/2021. Arthritis & Rheumatology. (2016).

Rath, Linda. "About Arthritis." https://www.arthritis.org/about-arthritis. Arthritis Foundation. (2022).

4
PART

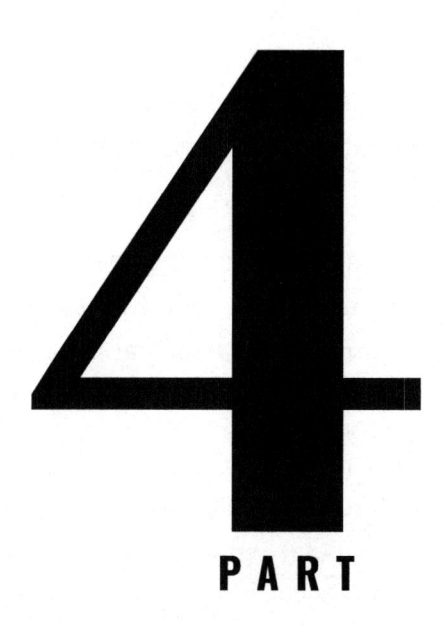

Arthritis Cookbook

EASY AND TASTY RECIPES

When starting a new way of eating, it's helpful to start with a positive mindset. Be open to trying new ingredients, and treat each new recipe as an adventure. To get motivated, remind yourself that you're making food that can reduce inflammation which will help ease your symptoms of arthritis.

With the master shopping list included in the next section, you'll know all the ingredients needed to make every recipe in this cookbook. The ingredients are available at a typical grocery store or supermarket, and many might already be in your pantry.

The recipes can be adapted to a casual way of cooking, that is, while you should measure some ingredients such as baking powder, you can use a freer hand with other ingredients such as blueberries and spinach. Please feel free to adapt, according to your preferences.

The Recipes

Breakfast

- Oatmeal Berry Bowl with Nuts and Oranges
- Triple Yum Yogurt with Muesli, Nuts, and Berries
- Oat and Banana Pancakes
- Breakfast Burrito

Lunch

- Tuna Salad with Leafy Greens and Fresh Vegetables
- Grain and Veggie "Buddha" Bowl
- Penne Pasta with Tomato and Grilled Green Vegetables
- Pitas with Falafels and Hummus
- Butternut Squash Soup

Dinner

- Baked Salmon with Fresh and Savory Green Vegetables
- Baked Chicken with Red Peppers and Sweet Potato
- Creamy Avocado Pasta with Green Beans and Cabbage
- Vegetable or Chicken Stir-Fry

Dessert

- Chocolate Chia Pudding with Blueberries
- Nut Butter Banana Smoothie

Master Shopping List

Fruit

- *Bananas*
- *Blueberries*
- *Oranges*
- *Strawberries*
- *Alternative fruit suggestions: pineapple and grapes*

Vegetables

- *Avocado*
- *Baby corn*
- *Broccoli*
- *Butternut squash*
- *Cabbage (red and white shredded)*
- *Carrots*
- *Cherry tomatoes*
- *Cucumber*
- *Garlic*
- *Ginger*
- *Green beans*
- *Leafy greens*
- *Lemons*
- *Onion*
- *Red pepper*
- *Spinach*
- *Sweet potato*

Dairy

- *Greek yogurt*
- *Oat milk (or plant-based milk of choice)*

Nuts and Seeds

- *Almonds*
- *Chia seeds*
- *Sesame*
- *Walnuts*

Grains

- *Oats*
- *Muesli (low sugar)*
- *Couscous*
- *Pita Bread, whole wheat*
- *Penne pasta (gluten-free)*
- *Rice noodles*
- *Tortillas, whole wheat*

Canned/Packaged Goods

- Black olives
- Chickpeas
- Falafel
- Tuna

Poultry/Fish

- Eggs
- Chicken filet
- Salmon filet

Spices, Flavorings, and Condiments

- Baking powder
- Cacao powder
- Chili flakes
- Cinnamon, ground
- Cumin
- Garlic powder
- Honey
- Olive oil
- Pepper
- Salt
- Soy sauce
- Vanilla extract
- Vegetable bouillon cubes

Helpful kitchen tools to have on hand

- Bullet mixer or blender
- Stick blender
- Kitchen scale to measure portions
- Sauté pans, small and large
- Medium pot
- Grater
- Foil to cover baking sheets
- _____
- _____
- _____
- _____
- _____
- _____
- _____
- _____

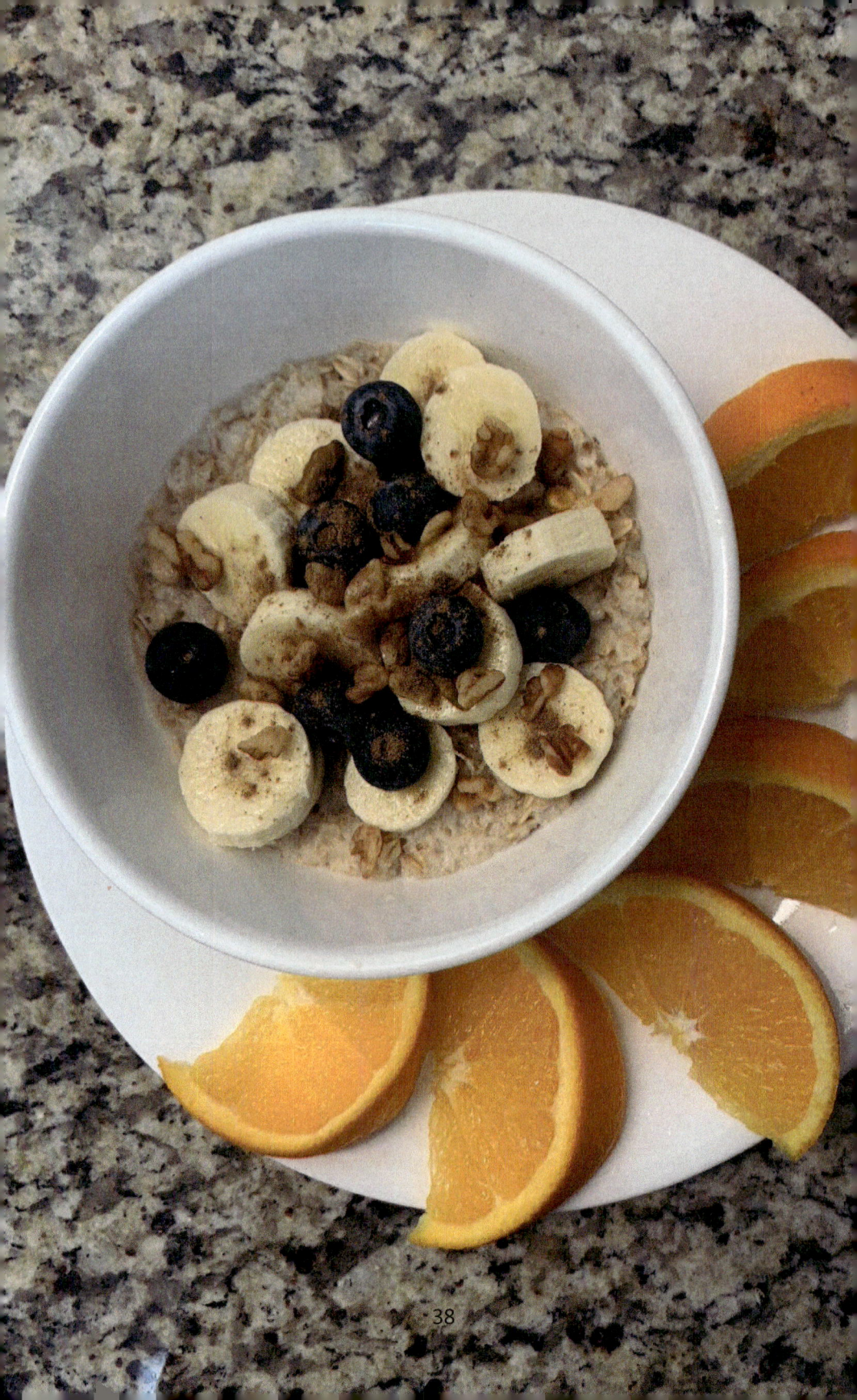

Oatmeal Berry Bowl with Nuts and Orange Slices

Cooking Time: 15 min   **Serves: 1**

Oatmeal with berries, banana, walnuts, a sprinkle of cinnamon, and a side of sliced oranges.

A high-fiber breakfast full of healthy, anti-inflammatory ingredients; high in vitamin C and omega-3 fatty acids.

Ingredients

- ½ cup oats (45 g)
- 1 banana, small
- About 8 blueberries (20 g)
- ¼ cup walnuts, chopped (15 g)
- ¼ teaspoon cinnamon, ground
- 1 orange, medium

> **Nutrition**
> Calories: 346;
> Carbohydrates: 50g;
> Sugar: 15g;
> Fiber: 8g;
> Fat: 13g;
> Protein: 8g;
> Sodium: 3mg

Directions

1. Place oats into a pot, add 1 cup cold water and bring to a boil; lower heat and simmer for 5 minutes. Scoop cooked oatmeal into a bowl.
2. Wash blueberries.
3. Slice banana and place on top of cooked oatmeal.
4. Add blueberries and chopped walnuts.
5. Sprinkle with cinnamon.
6. Slice orange and serve on the side.

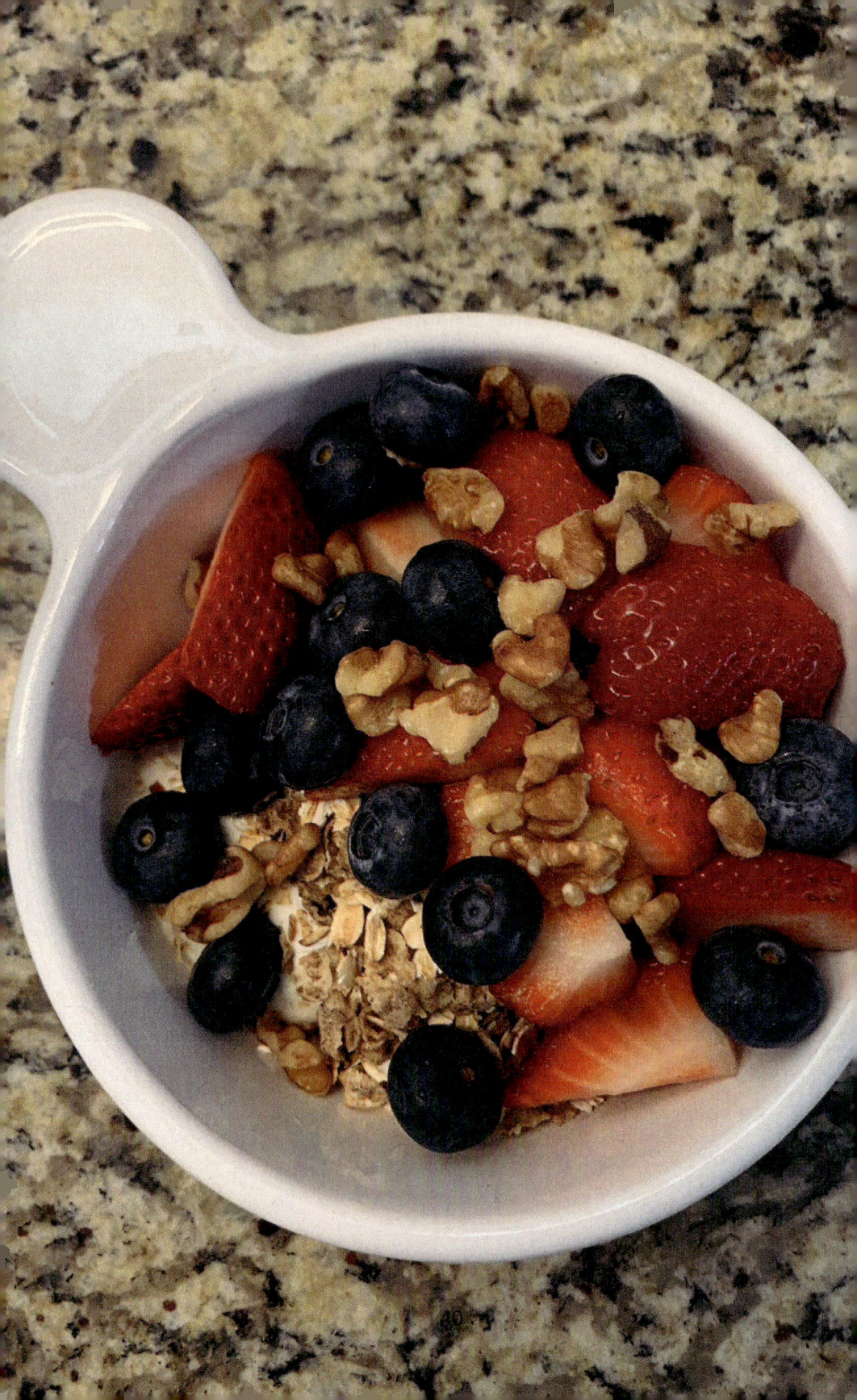

Triple Yum Yogurt with
Muesli, Nuts, and Berries

Cooking Time: 15 min   Serves: 1

Greek yogurt with muesli, walnuts, strawberries, and blueberries. An anti-inflammatory breakfast loaded with protein, gut-loving fiber, probiotics, vitamin C, and healthy omega-3 fatty acids.

Ingredients

- 4 heaping tablespoons Greek yogurt (80 g)
- ⅓ cup muesli, low sugar (45 g)
- About 4-6 strawberries (20 g)
- About 10-15 blueberries (20 g)
- ¼ cup walnuts (15 g)
- **Alternative fruit suggestions:** banana, pineapple, grapes, or oranges

Nutrition
Calories: 387;
Carbohydrates: 47g;
Sugar: 19g;
Fiber: 7g;
Fat: 18g;
Protein: 10g;
Sodium: 60mgg

Directions

1. Place Greek yogurt into a bowl.
2. Add muesli.
3. Rinse strawberries and blueberries well.
4. Cut strawberries into quarters and add to yogurt and muesli mix.
5. Add blueberries to yogurt and muesli mix.
6. Top with walnuts

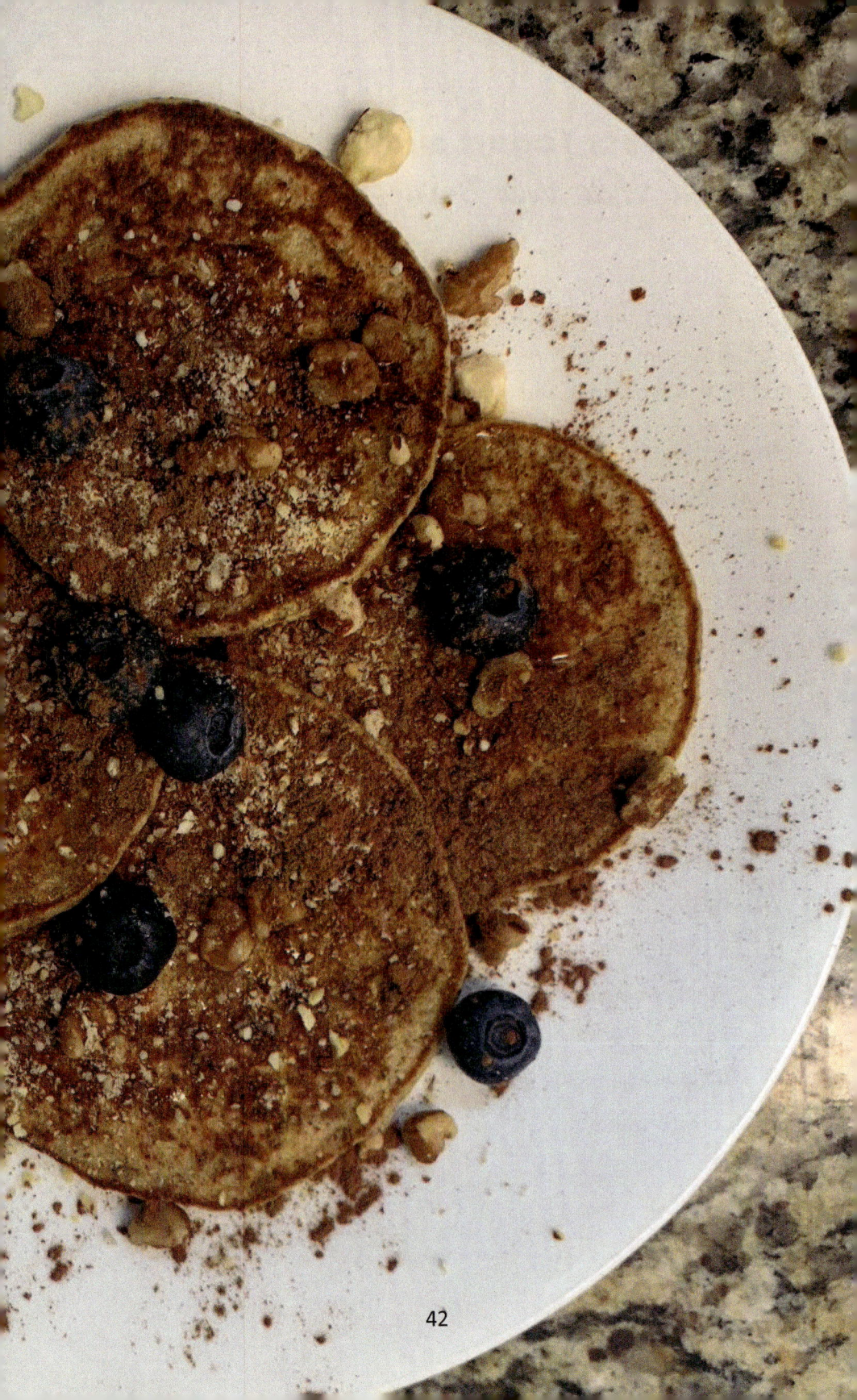

Oat and Banana Pancakes

Cooking Time: 20 min   Serves: 1 (4 pancakes)

Delicious and moist gluten-free pancakes topped with inflammation-fighting plant-foods: blueberries, cinnamon, cacao powder, walnuts, and almonds. A good source of protein, thiamine, riboflavin, vitamin B-6, magnesium, iron and selenium.

Ingredients

To make pancakes:

- 1 cup oats
- 1 medium ripe banana
- About ½ cup oat milk (or plant-based milk of choice)
- ½ tablespoon chia seeds
- 1 tablespoon honey
- 1 egg
- 1 teaspoon baking powder
- 1 teaspoon olive oil

Serve with:

- About 9 blueberries (.5 oz)
- ⅛ cup walnuts (.25 oz)
- ⅛ cup almonds (.25 oz)
- 1 teaspoon honey
- ¼ teaspoon cacao powder
- ¼ teaspoon cinnamon

> **Nutrition**
> Calories 719;
> Carbohydrates 110g;
> Sugar 234g;
> Fiber 20g;
> Fat 27g;
> Protein 27g;
> Sodium 212 mg

Directions

1. Using a stick blender or bullet mixer, blend oats for 30 seconds until fine.
2. Mash banana with fork and place into blender or bullet mixer.
3. Add the remaining ingredients (oat milk, chia seeds, baking powder, egg, and honey) to the blender.
4. Process until mixture is well-combined and smooth.
5. Add 1 tablespoon of olive oil to a frying pan and heat at medium heat.
6. Using a ladle, place 4 equal spoonfuls of batter into the pan.
7. After bubbles begin to form on pancake, gently flip over and cook until golden brown.
8. Place pancakes onto a plate and spread with honey.
9. Crush walnuts and almonds and sprinkle onto pancakes.
10. Top with blueberries.
11. Sprinkle with cacao powder and cinnamon.

Note:

Recipe makes about 6 pancakes (5-inch), so you can freeze 2 for later. If you prefer, substitute 4 store-bought pancakes (gluten-free).

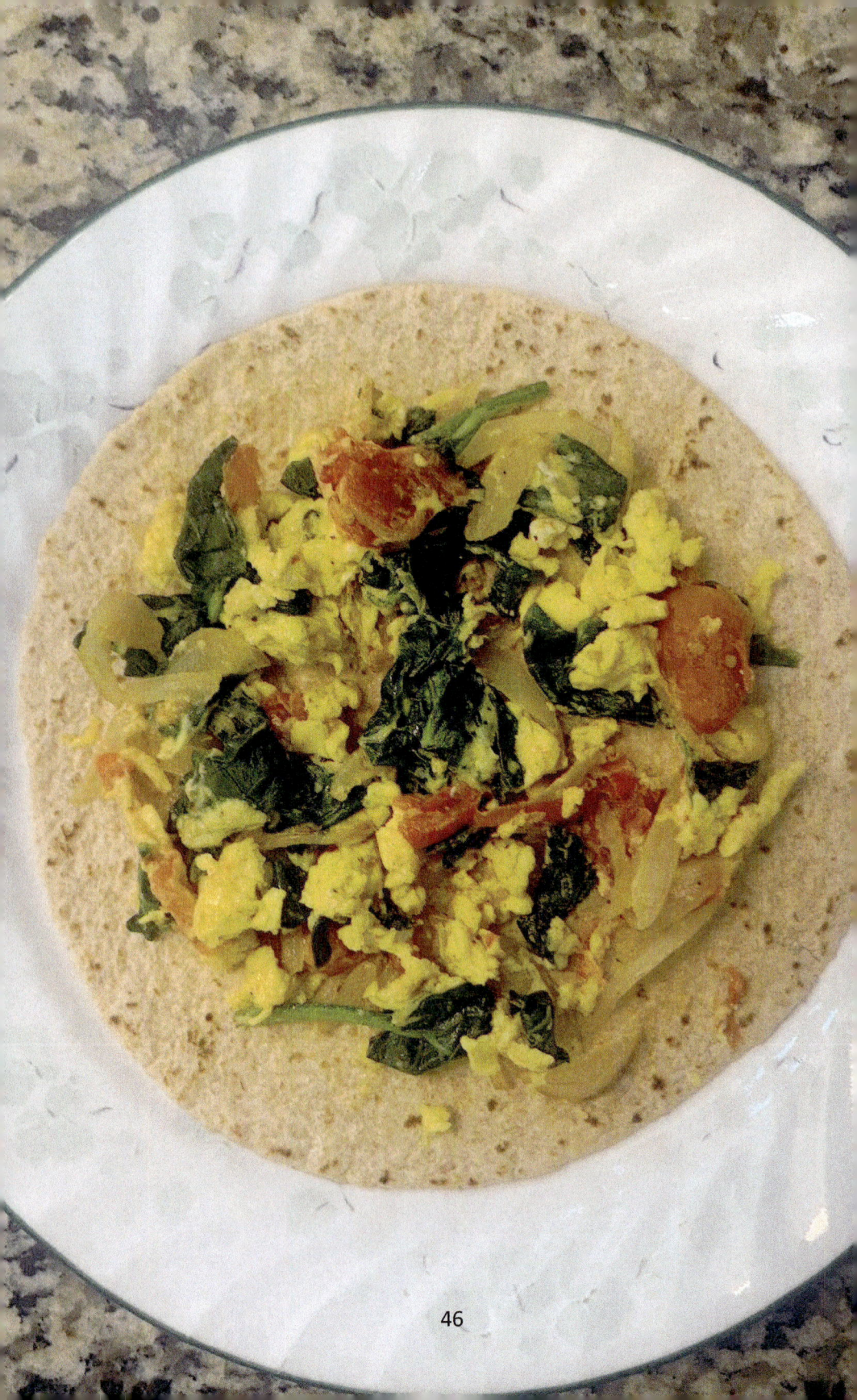

Breakfast Burrito

Cooking Time: 15 min **Serves: 1**

A warm breakfast burrito filled with egg, spinach, tomato, and onion. A good source of protein, riboflavin (vitamin B2), iron, and selenium. High in vitamins A and K.

Ingredients

- 1 medium whole-wheat tortilla
- 1 egg
- About 1 cup spinach (1 oz)
- About 4 cherry tomatoes (1 oz)
- 1/4 onion (.5 oz)
- 1 teaspoon olive oil
- Salt and pepper

Nutrition
Calories 177;
Carbohydrates 19g;
Sugar 3g;
Fiber 2g;
Fat 7g;
Protein 10g;
Sodium 309 mg

Directions

1. Crack egg into a bowl, and lightly beat. Add a pinch of salt and pepper to the mixture.
2. Wash spinach and tomatoes.
3. Chop spinach into smaller pieces.
4. Slice tomato and onion into smaller pieces.
5. Heat a pan over medium heat, and pour 1 teaspoon of olive oil into the pan.
6. Add tomato and onion and cook for 5 minutes.

7. Add spinach and cook for another minute.
8. Pour egg over the cooked vegetables, and stir the mixture until egg is cooked.
9. Heat tortilla on a separate pan for 30 seconds.
10. Place tortilla onto plate and fill with egg mixture; fold into burrito.

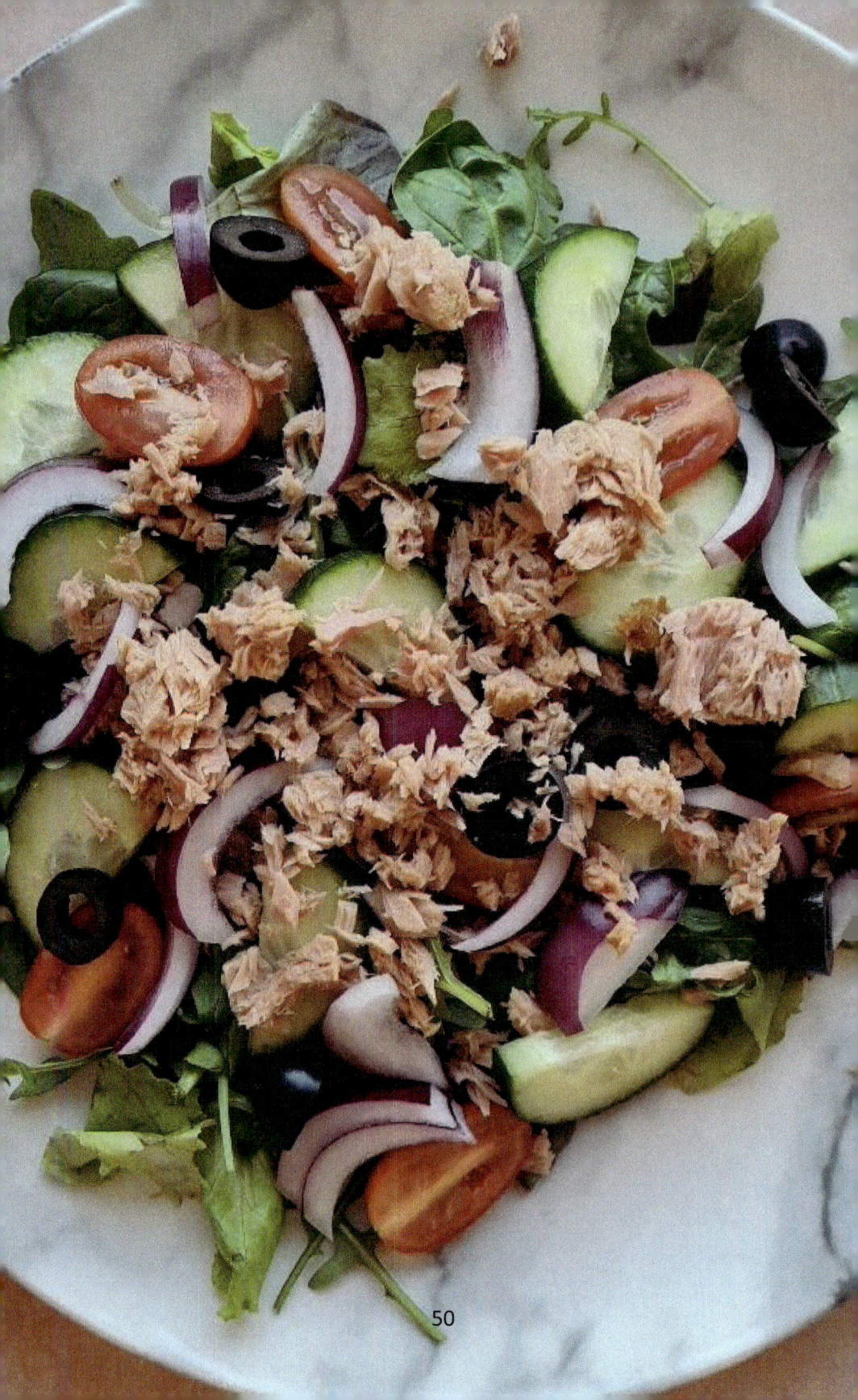

Tuna Salad with Leafy Greens & Fresh Vegetables

Cooking Time: 20 min **Serves: 1**

Tuna on a bed of leafy greens, with red onion, cherry tomatoes, cucumber, and black olives. An incredibly healthy lunch, loaded with a range of anti-inflammatory ingredients high in vitamins B3, B12, A, K, and selenium.

Ingredients

- 3 oz can of tuna (80 g)
- About 1 cup leafy greens (50 g)
- About 4 cherry tomatoes (50 g)
- About ½ cucumber (50 g)
- About ⅓ onion (30 g)
- About 4 black olives (20 g)
- 2 teaspoons olive oil
- Salt and pepper

> **Nutrition**
> Calories: 215;
> Carbohydrates: 9g;
> Sugar: 4g;
> Fiber: 3g;
> Fat: 13g;
> Protein: 17g;
> Sodium: 354mg

Directions

1. Wash leafy greens, and place them onto a plate.
2. Wash tomatoes and cucumber.
3. Cut cucumber and tomatoes into halves; place on top of leafy greens.
4. Cut olives into slices, and place on top of the salad.
5. Cut red onion into slices and place on top of salad.
6. Open can of tuna and drain; separate half the tuna and place on top of salad.
7. Drizzle salad with olive oil; add salt and pepper to taste.

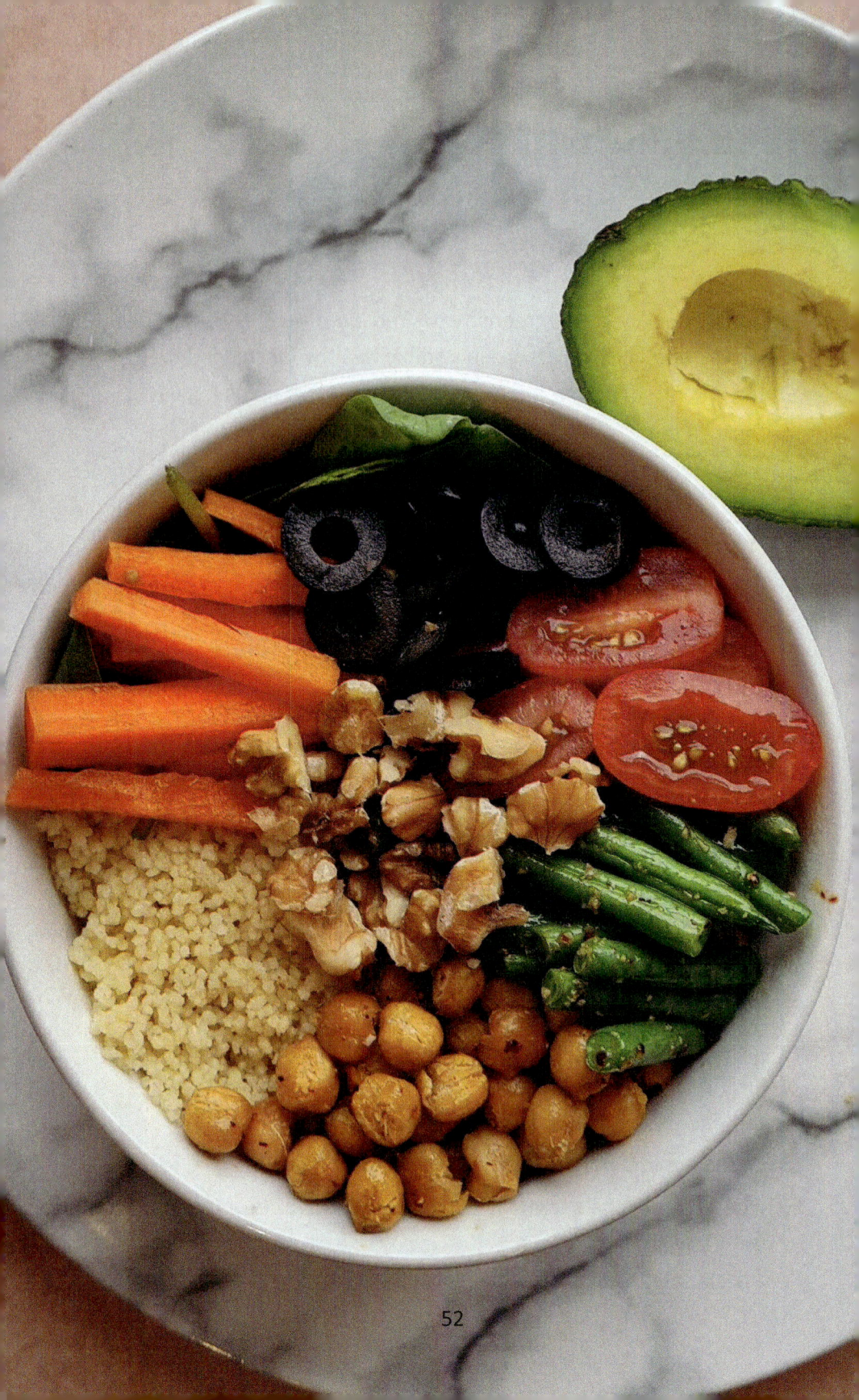

Grain and Veggie *"Buddha" Bowl*

Cooking Time: 30 min   Serves: 1

Oven-roasted chickpeas marinated in cumin and olive oil, served with couscous, green beans, cherry tomatoes, black olives, grated carrots, and avocado, then drizzled with olive oil and topped with crushed walnuts. A high-protein meal, full of healthy anti-inflammatory ingredients, high in vitamin A, iron, and omega-3 fatty acids.

Ingredients

- ½ cup chickpeas, canned (120 g)
- ½ cup couscous (60 g)
- About 10 green beans (25 g)
- About 5 cherry tomatoes (20 g)
- Carrot, small (30 g)
- ½ cup spinach (20 g)
- Avocado, small (40 g)
- About 4 Black olives (20 g)
- ¼ cup walnuts, chopped (15 g)
- 3 teaspoons olive oil
- ¼ teaspoon cumin
- ½ teaspoon garlic powder

> **Nutrition**
> Calories: 902;
> Carbohydrates: 92g;
> Sugar: 9g;
> Fiber: 19g;
> Fat: 51g;
> Protein: 23g;
> Sodium: 210mg

Directions

1. Preheat oven to 350°F (180°C).
2. Drain and rinse chickpeas.

3. Place chickpeas on a baking sheet and lightly drizzle with olive oil, cumin, and ¼ teaspoon garlic powder.
4. Place sheet in preheated oven for 20 minutes, until chickpeas become golden brown.
5. Boil water for couscous. Use 1 part boiled water (½ cup) to 1 part couscous (½ cup) and allow to sit for 5 minutes. Once water is absorbed, drizzle with olive oil, salt and pepper to taste.
6. Wash green beans, tomatoes, carrot, and spinach well.
7. Cut green beans into thirds and sauté in a pan containing 1 teaspoon olive oil and remaining ¼ teaspoon garlic powder at medium heat for 5 minutes.
8. Peel carrot and cut into small pieces.
9. Cut cherry tomatoes and olives into slices.
10. Place spinach in bottom of bowl.
11. Add cooked couscous and roasted chickpeas and the rest of the vegetables: carrots, olives, tomatoes, and sautéed green beans.
12. Top with walnuts.
13. Drizzle with olive oil.
14. Cut avocado into slices and serve on the side.

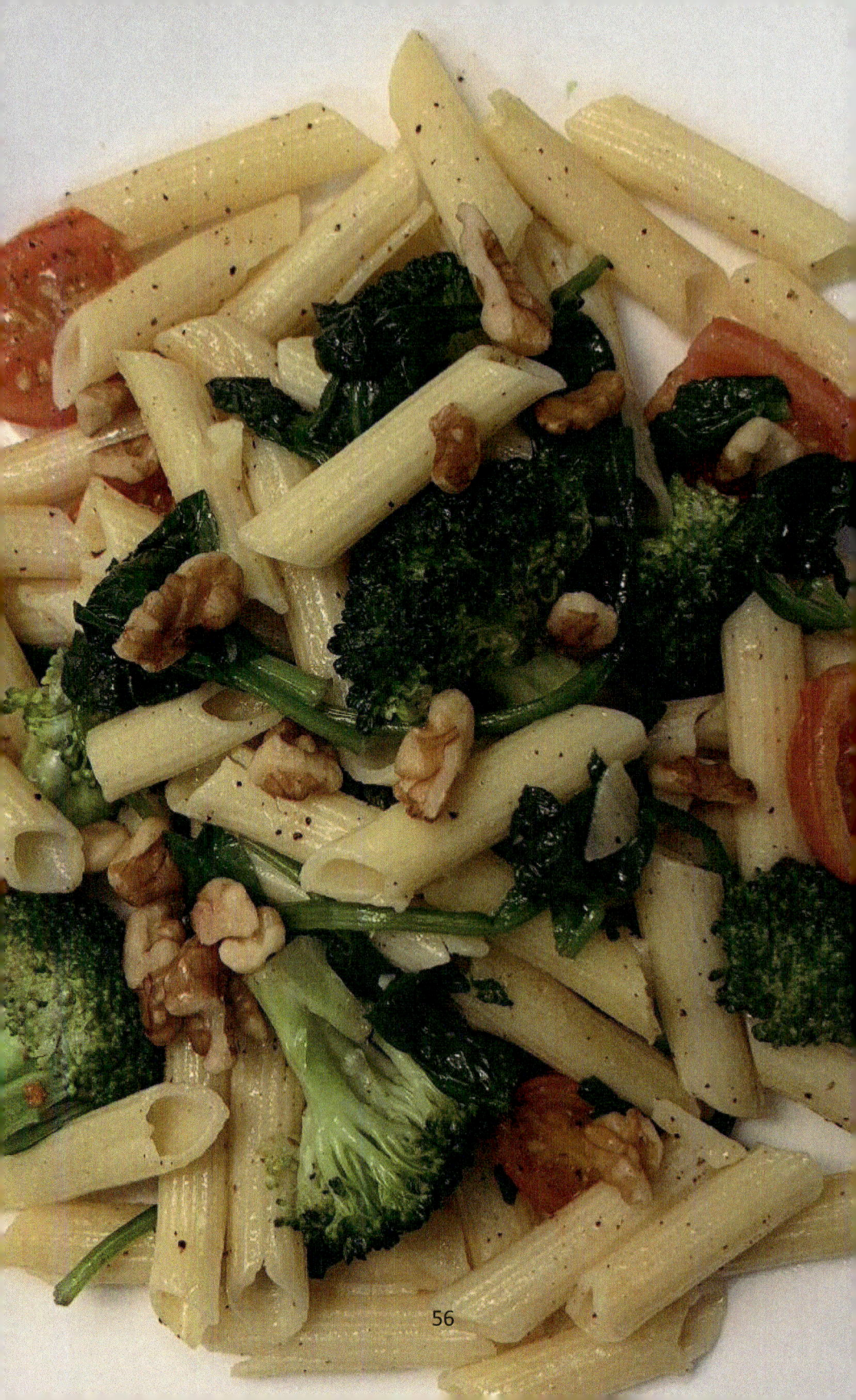

Penne Pasta with Tomato & Grilled Green Vegetables

Cooking Time: 35 min   **Serves:** 1

Gluten-free penne pasta, with a tomato, garlic, and olive oil base, topped with broccoli and spinach, and sprinkled with chopped walnuts. A delicious and easy lunch to prepare, full of healthy anti-inflammatory ingredients, high in omega-3 fatty acids, vitamins C, A, and K, and iron.

Ingredients

- ¾ cup gluten-free penne pasta (75 g)
- About 5 broccoli florets (60 g)
- About 2 cups spinach (50 g)
- About 4 cherry tomatoes (50 g)
- ¼ cup walnuts, chopped (15 g)
- 2 tablespoons olive oil, plus more for drizzling
- Chili flakes, pinch (or as preferred)
- ¼ teaspoon garlic powder
- Salt and pepper

Nutrition
Calories: 661;
Carbohydrates: 71g;
Sugar: 3g;
Fiber: 7g;
Fat: 38g;
Protein: 12g;
Sodium: 332mg

Directions

1. Bring a medium pot of water to a boil; add pasta and simmer for 20 minutes.
2. Wash and cut broccoli. Add to a pan and sauté at medium heat with 1 tablespoon of olive oil, a pinch of chili flakes, and salt and pepper to taste; cook until broccoli becomes soft, stirring occasionally.

3. Wash spinach, and place in the same pan as broccoli. Place a lid on the pan to allow the spinach to wilt slightly.

4. In a separate pot, add cherry tomatoes, 1 tablespoon of olive oil, garlic powder, and a pinch of pepper. Cook at medium heat for 5 minutes, until tomatoes become soft.

5. Once pasta is cooked al dente, drain and allow to stand for 2 minutes.

6. Place pasta back in pot, drizzle with olive oil, and add salt and pepper to taste.

7. Place pasta on plate, then add cooked tomatoes, broccoli, and spinach; sprinkle with walnuts.

60

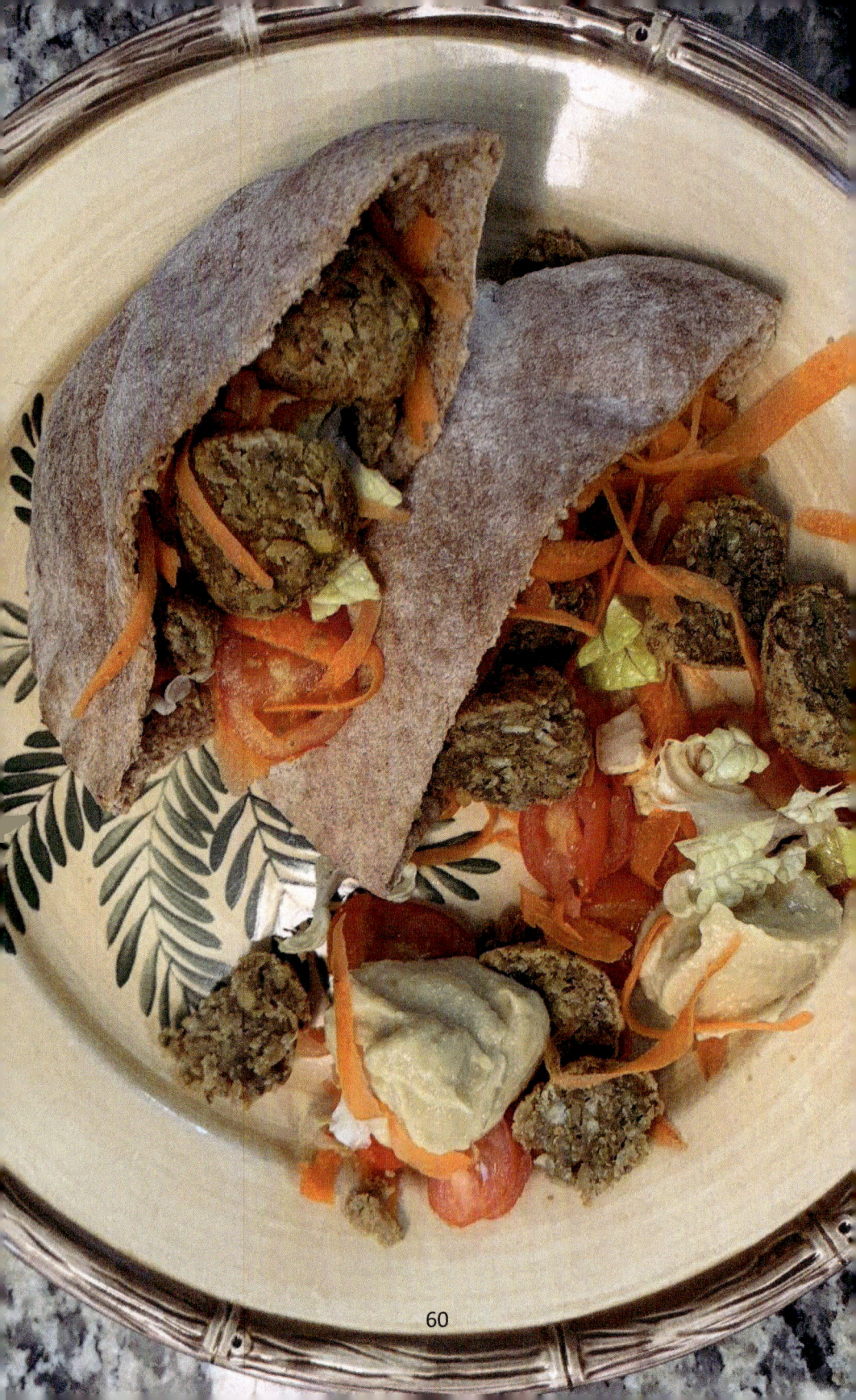

Pitas with Falafels and Hummus

Cooking Time: 20 min **Serves:** 1

A tasty whole-wheat pita bread with hummus, falafels, shredded carrots, cabbage, and tomatoes. Source of protein, vitamin B6, iron, and selenium. High in vitamin A.

Ingredients

- 1 whole-wheat pita bread
- 4-5 falafels, store-bought (1.76 oz.)
- 2 tablespoons hummus, plain
- 1 carrot, small (.88 oz)
- ½ cup cabbage, shredded (.88 oz)
- 2 cherry tomatoes (.70 oz.)
- 1 onion, small (0.50 oz.)

Nutrition
Calories 417;
Carbohydrates 63g;
Sugar 5g;
Fiber 14g;
Fat 13g;
Protein 15g;
Sodium 450mg

Directions

1. Cut pita bread in half and toast each half in toaster or oven.
2. Prepare falafels. Follow package directions to cook. If fully cooked, warm in microwave or oven.
3. Wash carrot and tomatoes.
4. Slice tomatoes.
5. Grate carrot until finely shredded.
6. Cut onion into slices.
7. Fill each pita bread half with shredded cabbage, grated carrot, tomato, and onion.
8. Add 2-3 falafels into each pita half.
9. Serve with hummus.

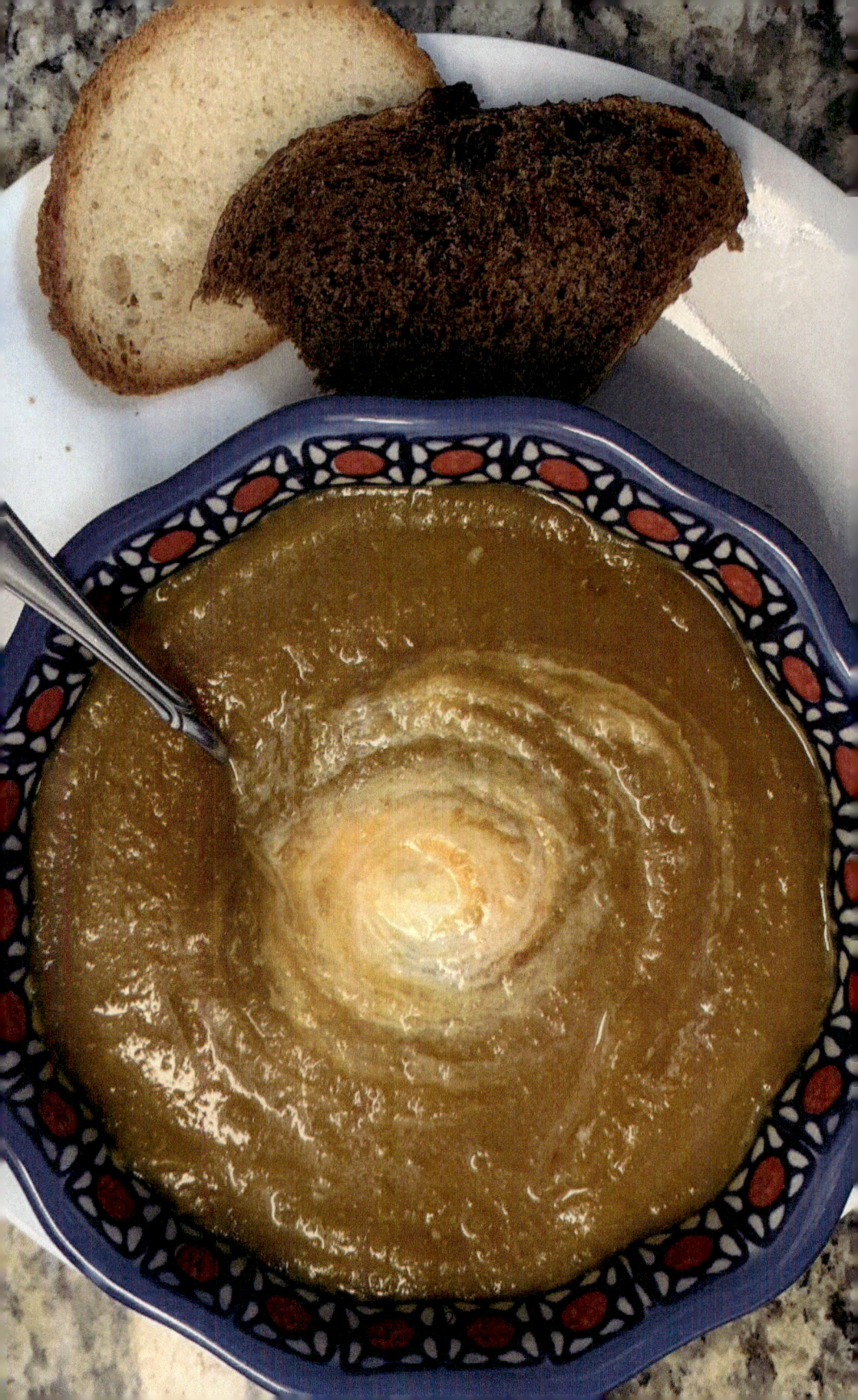

Butternut Squash Soup

Cooking Time: 60 min   Serves: 1

A hearty, warm butternut soup with a hint of chili; can be served with a dollop of Greek yogurt. High in vitamins A and C, and a source of potassium.

Ingredients

- About 2 cups butternut squash, cubed (8.80 oz)
- ½ onion, chopped (2 oz)
- 2 garlic cloves
- ½ vegetable bouillon cube
- 1 cup water (8 fl oz)
- ¼ tsp chili flakes
- Salt and pepper
- Greek yogurt (optional)

Nutrition
Calories 101;
Carbohydrates 27g;
Sugar 6g;
Fiber 9g;
Fat 13g;
Protein 2g;
Sodium 450mg

Directions

1. Place medium-sized pot on medium heat and add 1 tablespoon olive oil.
2. Chop onion and place into the pot to brown for 10 minutes.
3. Mince garlic cloves and place into the pot with onions. Add chili flakes. Sauté for 5 minutes.
4. Add cubed butternut to the pot and cover with 1 cup of water.
5. Add stock cube to the mixture. Stir well and cover with lid.
6. Allow to simmer for 20 minutes until soft.

7. Remove from heat and allow to cool for 10 minutes.
8. Using a stick blender, blend the mixture into a smooth consistency making sure all butternut is well blended.
9. Pour into a bowl.
10. Add salt and pepper to taste and a dollop of Greek yogurt (optional).
11. Serve with whole grain bread, such as rye or pumpernickel.

66

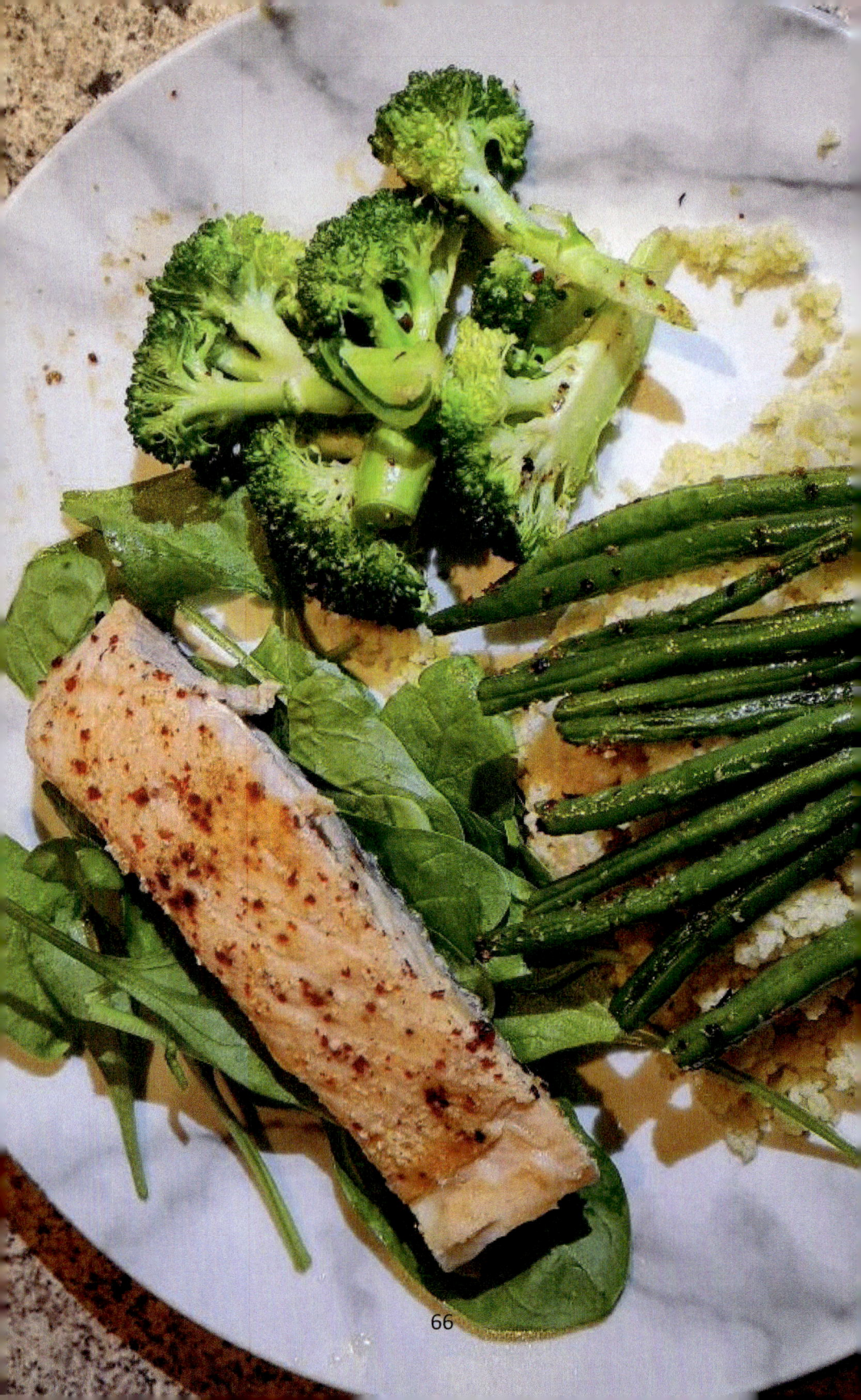

Baked Salmon with Fresh & Savory Green Vegetables

Cooking Time: 35 min Serves: 1

Baked salmon on a bed of spinach, with sautéed broccoli and green beans in garlic and olive oil, with a side of couscous. A high-protein meal with a powerhouse of anti-inflammatory ingredients; high in healthy omega-3 fatty acids, vitamin C, zinc, selenium, and vitamin A.

Ingredients

- 1 salmon filet (125 g)
- ¼ cup couscous (60 g)
- One handful spinach
- About 6 green beans (50 g)
- About 5 broccoli florets (50 g)
- 2 tablespoons olive oil, plus more for drizzling
- ½ teaspoon garlic powder
- Chili flakes, pinch
- Salt and pepper

Nutrition
Calories: 580;
Carbohydrates: 33g;
Sugar: 1g;
Fiber: 5g;
Fat: 34g;
Protein: 35g;
Sodium: 250mg

Directions

1. Preheat oven to 350°F (180°C).
2. Marinate salmon in 1 tablespoon olive oil, ¼ tsp garlic powder, a pinch of chili flakes, and salt and pepper to taste.
3. To boil water for couscous: add 1 part boiled water to 1 part couscous and allow to sit for 5 minutes. Once water is absorbed, drizzle with olive oil, and salt and pepper to taste.

4. Wrap salmon filet in foil and bake in oven for 20 minutes.
5. Wash spinach, broccoli, and green beans.
6. Sauté broccoli and green beans in a pan with ¼ tsp garlic powder and 1 tablespoon of olive oil until soft.
7. Place spinach on plate and top with cooked salmon.
8. Place couscous on the side, and top with green beans and broccoli.

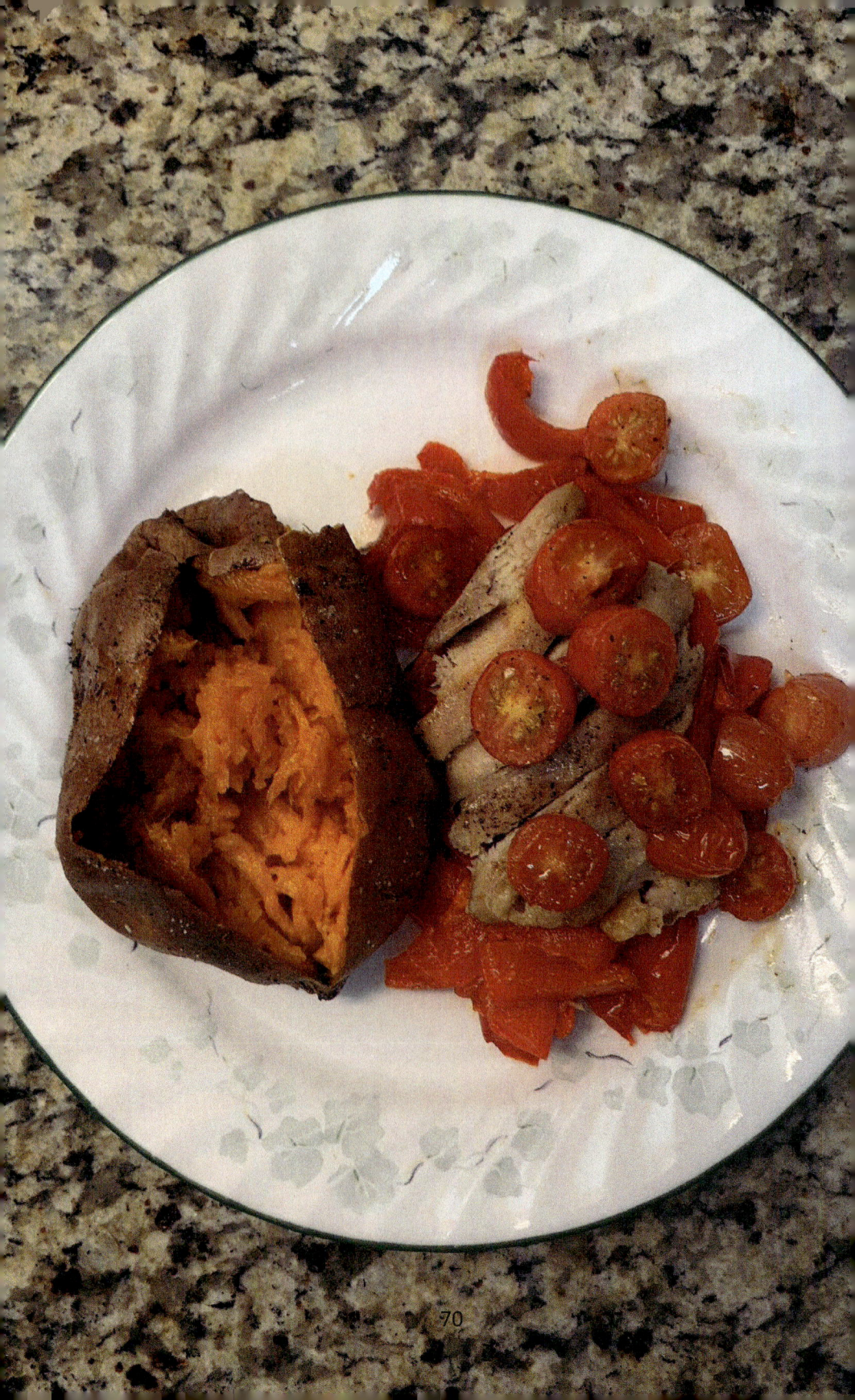

Baked Chicken with Red Peppers and Sweet Potato

Cooking Time: 60 min   Serves: 1

Baked chicken on a bed of roasted red pepper puree, topped with oven-roasted cherry tomatoes marinated in olive oil and pepper, served with a whole baked sweet potato. A delicious, high protein meal full of anti-inflammatory ingredients, high in vitamins A, E, B3, B6, and selenium.

Ingredients

- 1 chicken filet (150 g)
- 1 sweet potato, large
- ½ red pepper
- About 6 cherry tomatoes (50 g)
- 2 tablespoons olive oil, plus more for drizzling
- ½ teaspoon garlic powder, plus more for sprinkling
- Salt and pepper

Nutrition
Calories: 620;
Carbohydrates: 38g;
Sugar: 15g;
Fiber 3g;
Fat: 34g;
Protein: 41g;
Sodium: 80mg

Directions

1. Preheat oven to 350°F (180°C).
2. Marinate chicken filet in 1 tablespoon olive oil, ¼ tsp garlic powder, and salt and pepper to taste.
3. Wash sweet potato well and pierce all over with a fork.
4. Place sweet potato on a baking sheet covered with foil, and lightly drizzle with olive oil, and salt and pepper to taste. Place in oven and bake for 50-60 minutes, until easily pierced with a fork.

5. Wash red pepper, remove core, and cut into eighths. Season with olive oil and a sprinkle of garlic powder. Using another baking sheet covered with foil, place red pepper on one side.

6. Place chicken filet on other side of baking sheet; bake both for 30 minutes. Remove when done and cover to keep warm.

7. Wash cherry tomatoes, cut in halves, and place into a separate oven dish, lightly drizzle in olive oil, ¼ tsp of garlic powder, and salt and pepper to taste. Using the same baking sheet used for the chicken and red pepper, roast tomatoes in oven for 10 minutes.

8. Place red pepper on plate, followed by chicken filet; top with roasted cherry tomatoes. Cut cooked sweet potato in half and serve on the side.

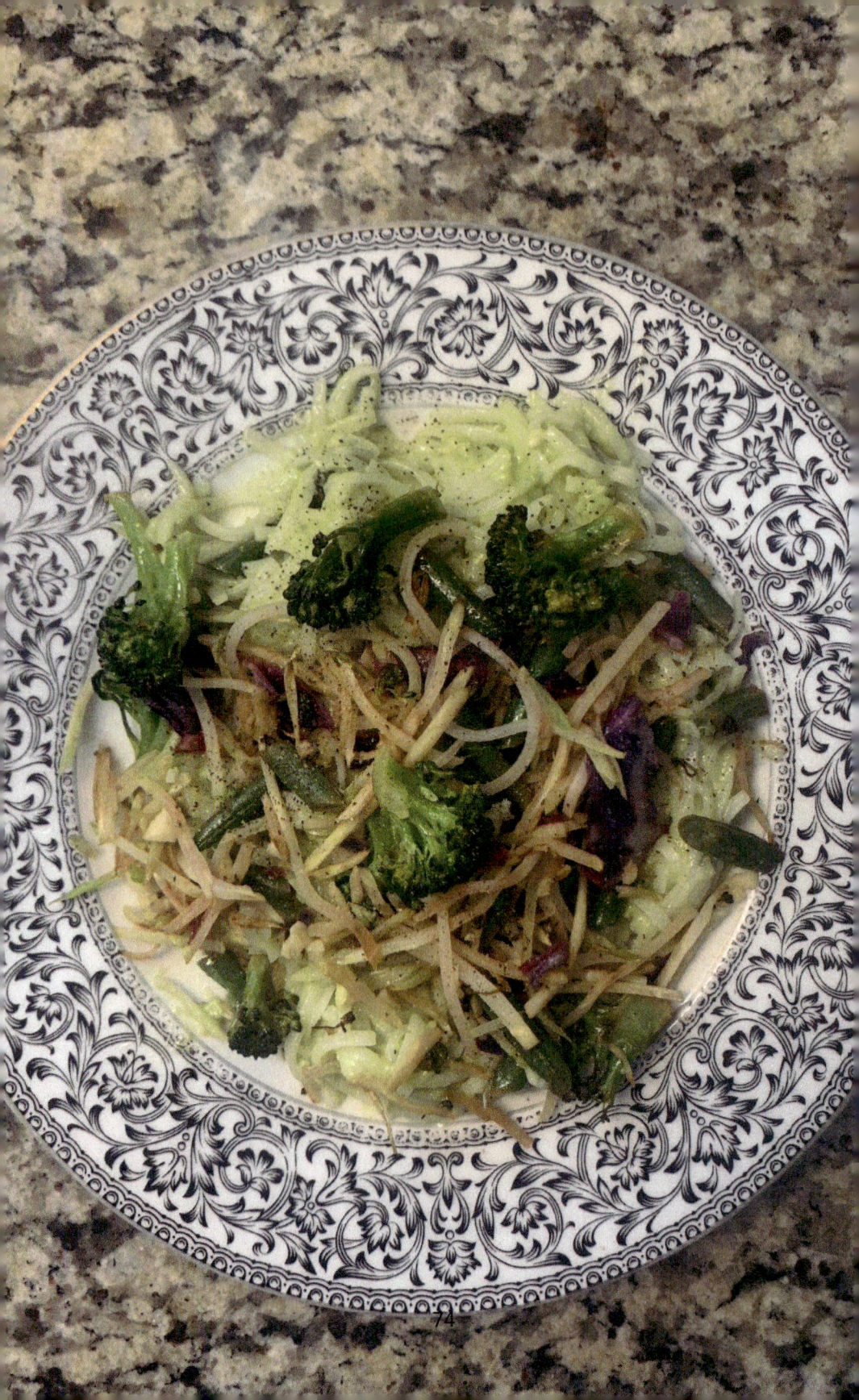

Creamy Avocado Pasta with Green Beans and Cabbage

Cooking Time: 45 min   Serves: 1

Creamy avocado pasta with broccoli, green beans, and red and white cabbage. A deliciously creamy, nutritious dinner full of anti-inflammatory ingredients. High in vitamins C, B6, A, E, K, folate, and iron.

Ingredients

- 3 oz gluten-free pasta
- About 1 cup red and white cabbage, shredded (2.5 oz)
- 1 avocado, small (2.3 oz)
- About 5 broccoli florets (1.76 oz)
- About 6 green beans (.88 oz)
- 2 garlic cloves, minced
- 3 tablespoons olive oil
- 1 teaspoon lemon juice
- Salt and pepper

Nutrition
Calories 708;
Carbohydrates 53g;
Sugar 4g;
Fiber 10g;
Fat 5g;
Protein 12g;
Sodium 200 mg

Directions

1. Bring a pot of water to boil; turn down heat to medium and place pasta into water. Simmer for about 10-15 minutes, until al dente.
2. Cut broccoli into small pieces about 1 inch in size.
3. Cut ends off of green beans and cut into 1 inch pieces.

4. Place pan over a medium heat, add 1 tablespoon olive oil, broccoli and green beans and sauté for 10 minutes until soft.
5. Wash cabbage well, place into pan with broccoli and green beans. Squeeze ¼ teaspoon lemon juice over the contents of the pan. Cover with lid and cook for 5 minutes.
6. Drain pasta, and allow to cool for 5 minutes.
7. Mash avocado with a fork.
8. Place pasta back into pot and drizzle generously with olive oil. Mix in the avocado.
9. Place avocado pasta onto a plate and top with the vegetable mix.

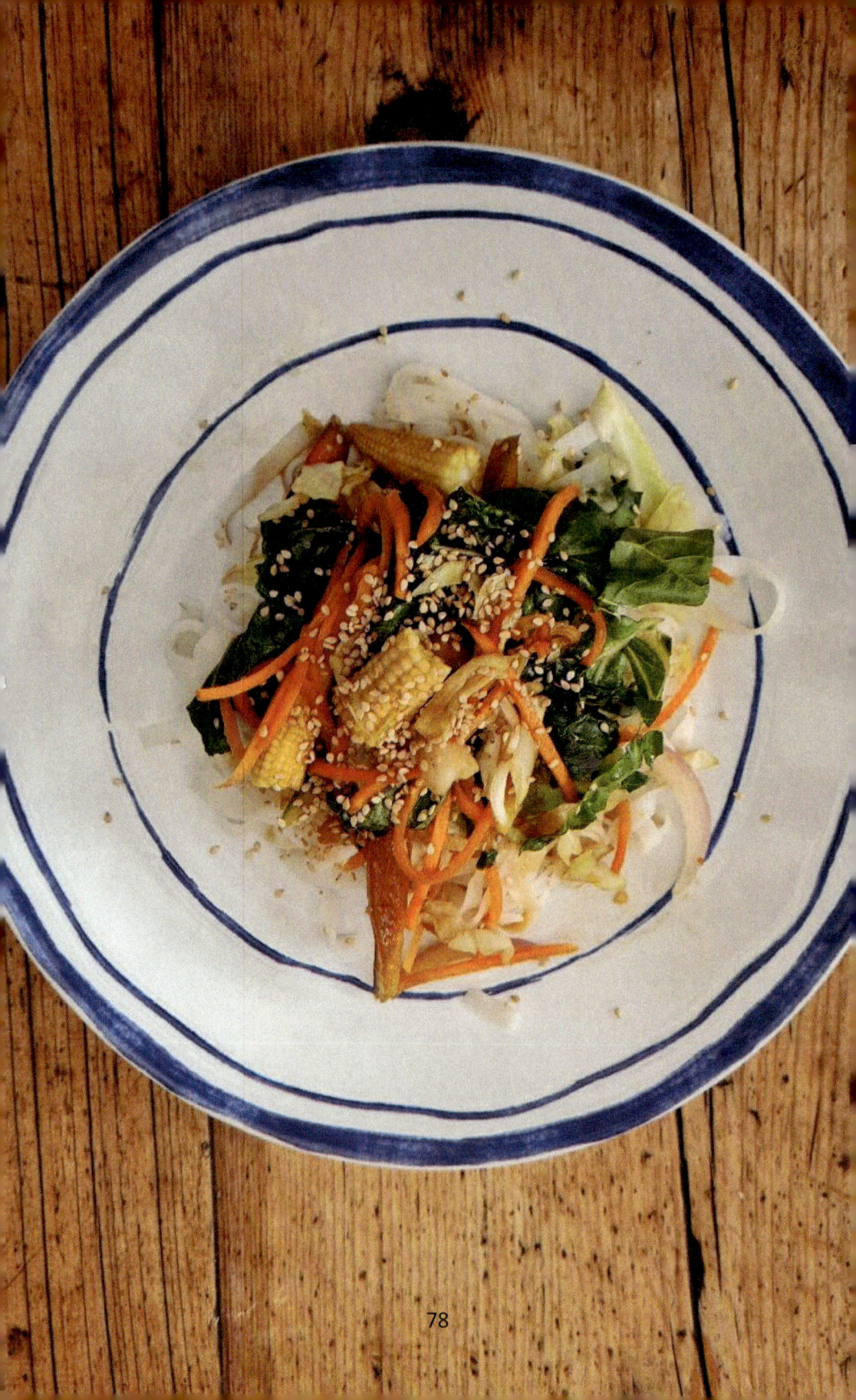

Vegetable Stir-Fry
– Chicken Stir-Fry

Cooking Time: 30 min **Serves: 1**

A fresh and crunchy vegetable stir-fry loaded with anti-inflammatory plant-foods to help alleviate the symptoms associated with arthritis. If desired, you can add chicken for additional protein. Each serving contains recommended daily amounts of vitamins A and K, B3, B6, selenium, and manganese.

Ingredients

- 3 oz. rice noodles
- *Stir-fry vegetables:
- 1 cup spinach
- ¼ cup baby corn
- 1 carrot, small
- 1/4 onion
- 2 tablespoons olive oil
- 2 tablespoons soy sauce
- 2 garlic cloves
- ½ inch ginger
- 1 teaspoon honey
- ¼ tsp chili flakes
- 1 teaspoon sesame seeds
- Salt and pepper

Nutrition (vegetarian)
Calories 511;
Carbohydrates 56g;
Sugar 9g;
Fiber 4g;
Fat 29g;
Protein 8g;
Sodium 1827 mg

Nutrition (with chicken)
Calories 601;
Carbohydrates 56g;
Sugar 9g;
Fiber 4g;
Fat 32g;
Protein 26g;
Sodium 1867 mg

Note:

A prepackaged stir-fry mix can be a convenient substitute for fresh vegetables; recipe uses about 3 oz, so you can save the rest for another meal. In some stir fry mixes, snow peas are substituted for baby corn.

To make stir-fry with chicken, add:

- 1 chicken filet (150 g)

Directions

1. Peel garlic and ginger root; cut into small pieces.
2. Wash vegetables.
3. Cut or tear spinach into pieces.
4. Peel carrot and shred into long, thin strips.
5. Remove onion skin and chop onion into pieces.
6. Cut tops off of baby corn and cut into 1 inch pieces.
7. Bring a medium-sized pan to medium-high heat; add olive oil. Place garlic, ginger, and chili flakes into the pan and cook for a few minutes.
8. Add vegetables and cook for 10 minutes, stirring regularly.
9. Pour in the soy sauce and honey, and cook for 5 more minutes. Set aside.
10. For the rice noodles, bring a medium-sized pot filled with water to boil. Reduce heat and add the rice noodles. Simmer for 5-10 minutes, until noodles are cooked through. Remove from heat and drain water.
11. Place noodles onto a plate, and top with the vegetable stir-fry mix.
12. Sprinkle with sesame seeds; add salt and pepper to taste.

Chicken option:

1. Cut chicken filet into pieces.
2. Heat a separate medium-sized pan to a medium heat. Pour in olive oil and cook chicken for 10-15 minutes, stirring occasionally until golden brown and cooked through.
3. Place cooked chicken on top of rice noodles and stir-fry vegetables.

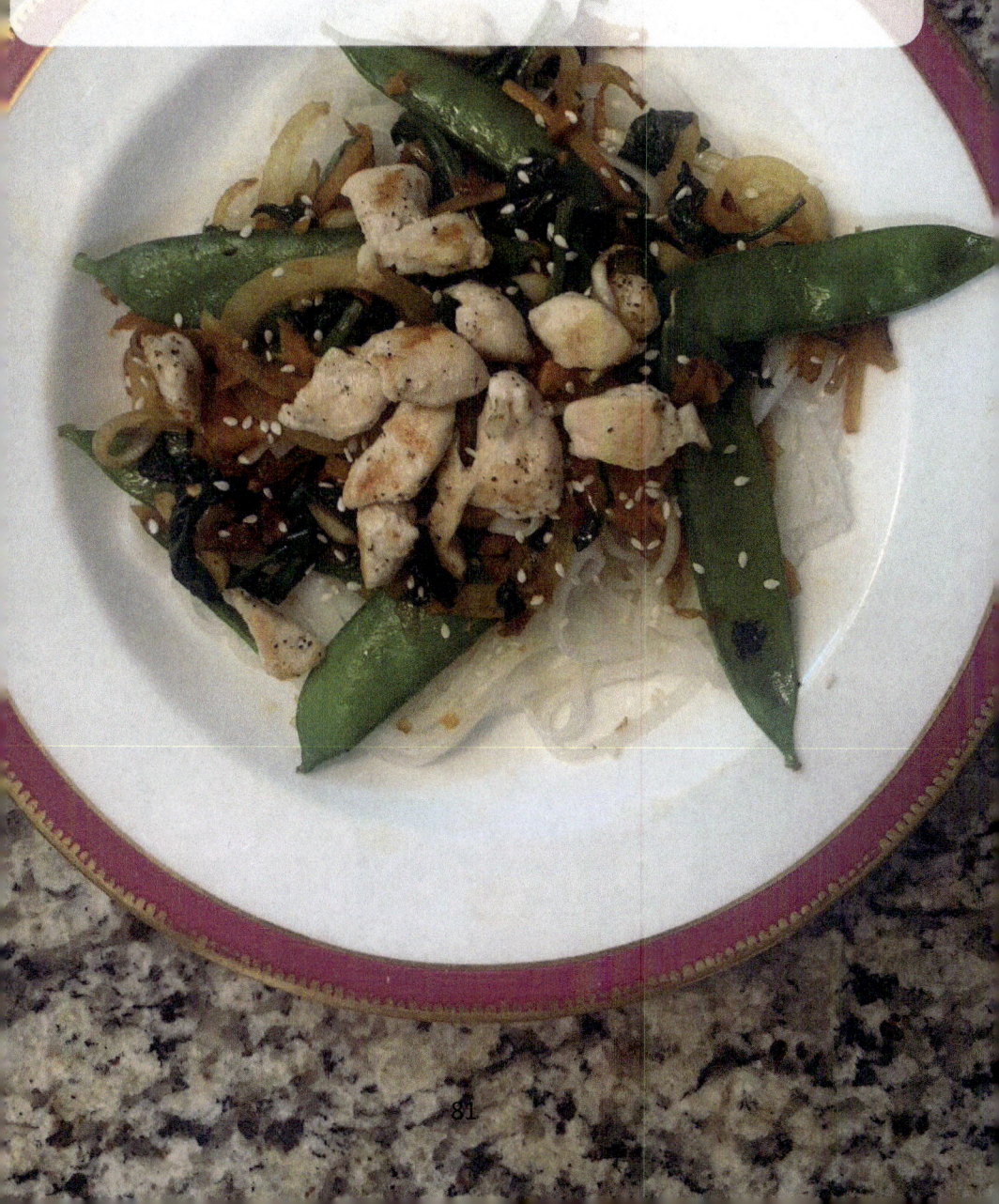

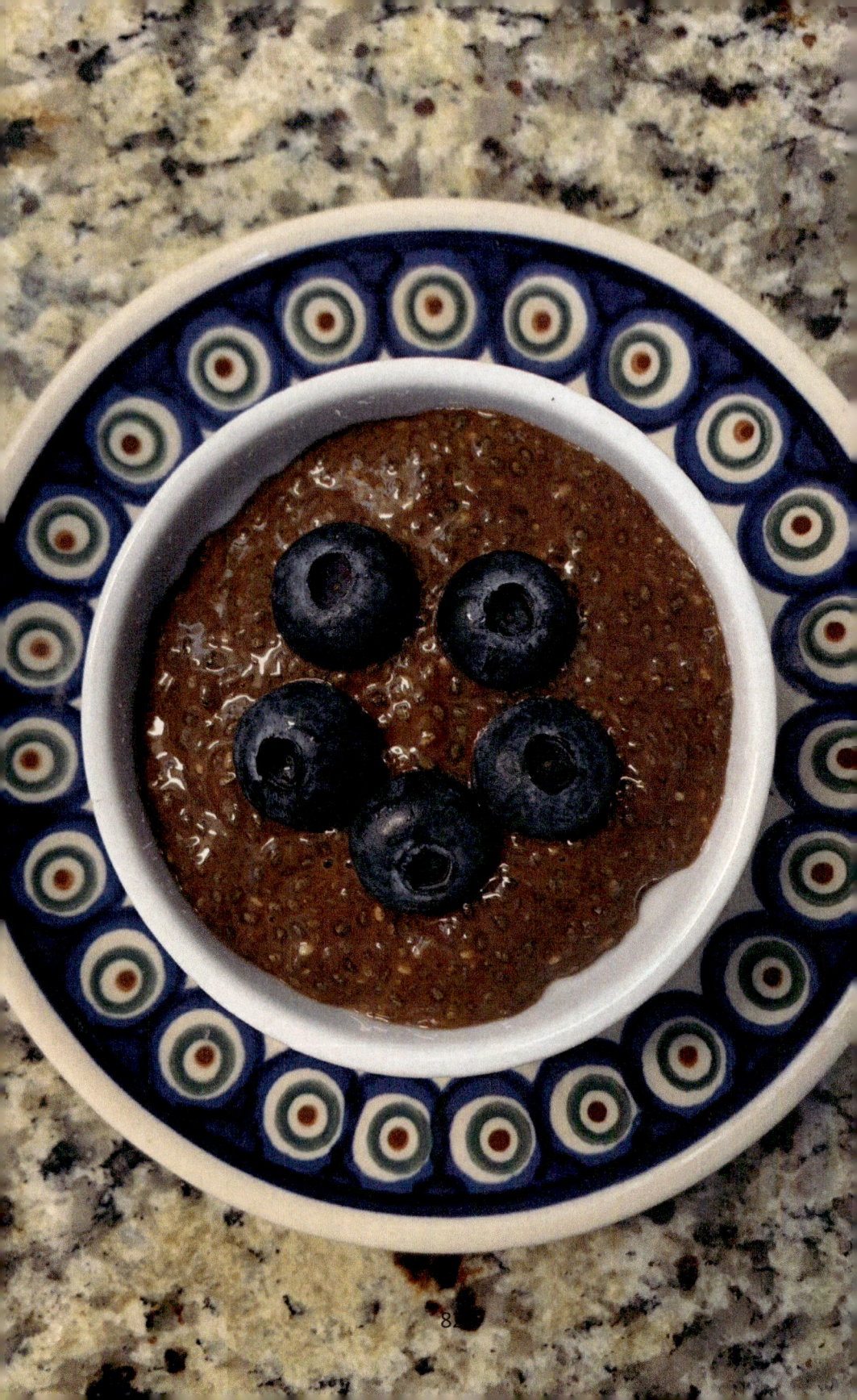

Chocolate Chia Pudding
with Blueberries

Prep time: 10 min + 2 hours in fridge to chill

Serves: 1

A tasty whole-wheat pita bread with hummus, falafels, shredded carrots, cabbage, and tomatoes. Source of protein, vitamin B6, iron, and selenium. High in vitamin A.

Ingredients

- 4 tablespoons chia seeds (1 oz)
- 1 tablespoon cacao powder (.18 oz)
- About ½ cup oat milk, or plant-based milk of choice (4.25 fl oz)
- 1 teaspoon honey
- About 5 blueberries (.35 oz)
- ¼ teaspoon cinnamon
- ¼ teaspoon vanilla extract

Nutrition
Calories 458;
Carbohydrates 28g;
Sugar 9g;
Fiber 13g;
Fat 14g;
Protein 7g;
Sodium 68 mg

Directions

1. Pour oat milk into bullet mixer or blender, followed by cacao powder, honey, cinnamon, and vanilla extract.
2. Blend for 15 seconds, until mixture is well-combined and there are no clumps.
3. Add chia seeds to the mixture and stir well.
4. Place mixture in the refrigerator for 2 hours.
5. After chilling, stir pudding well.
6. Spoon mixture into a small glass or bowl.
7. Add blueberries.

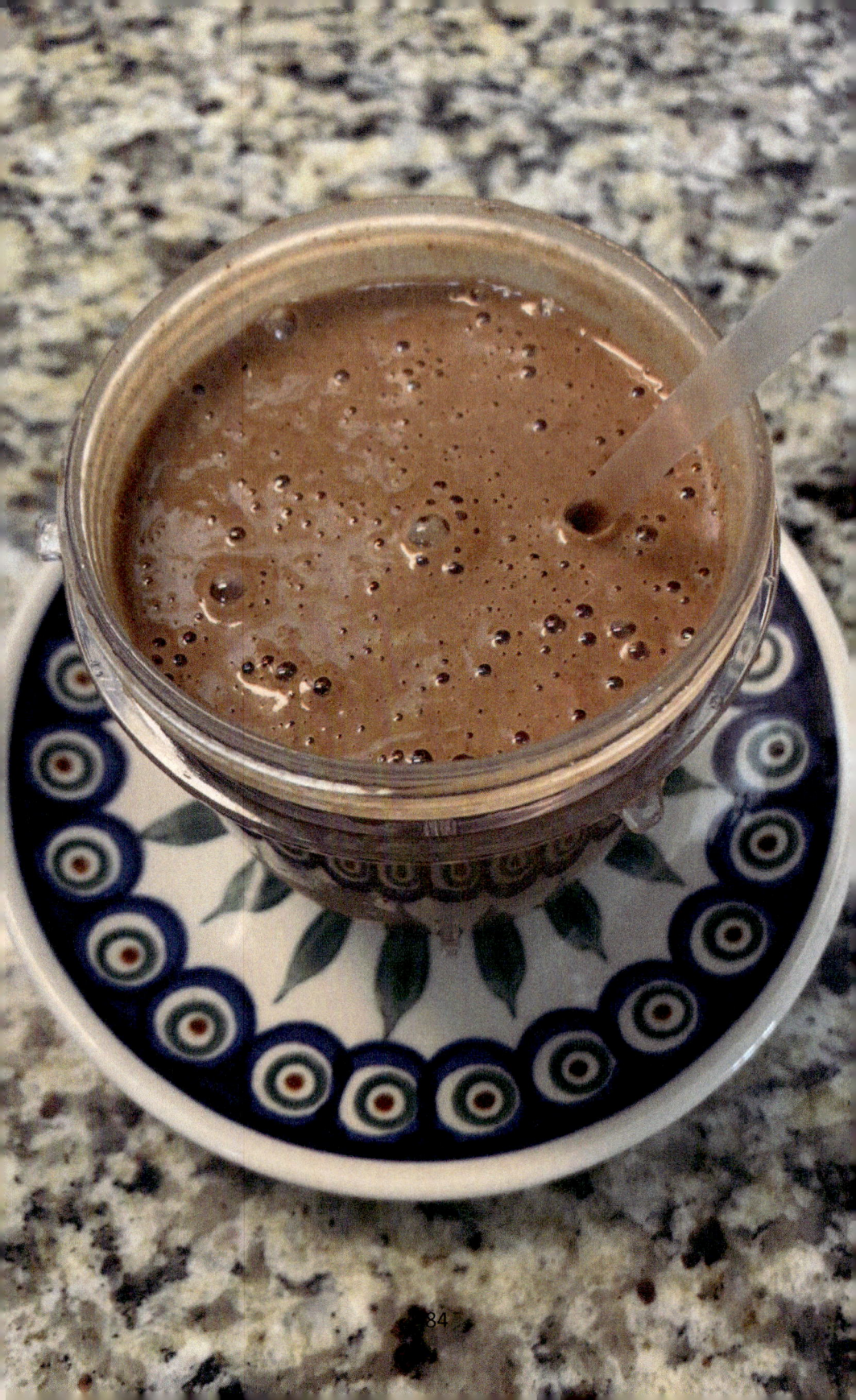

Nut Butter Banana Smoothie

Prep time: 5 min **Serves: 1**

An almond butter smoothie containing cacao powder, banana, and oat milk. This nourishing, delicious dessert is full of healthy fats, vitamins, minerals, and an anti-inflammatory powerhouse – cacao powder.

Ingredients

- 2 tablespoons almond butter, or nut butter of choice (1 oz)
- About ½ cup oat milk, or plant-based milk of choice (5 fl oz)
- 1 tablespoon cacao powder
- 1 banana, small (2.45 oz)

Nutrition
Calories 609;
Carbohydrates 34 g;
Sugar 16g
Fiber 8g;
Fat 23g;
Protein 9g;
Sodium 150mg

Directions

1. Place ingredients into a bullet mixer or blender.
2. Process on high for 30 seconds, until mixture is well combined and smooth.
3. Pour into a glass.

About the Author

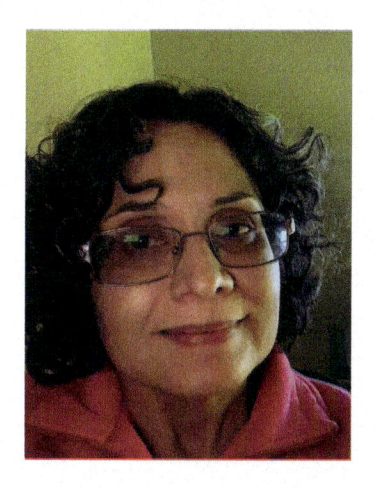

Libby Nau loves learning new things and working on projects that help people. She has a background in journalism, news reporting, editing, and self-publishing.

If you have any questions or want to contact Libby, please send an email to libby.aguigui.nau@gmail.com

Customer reviews

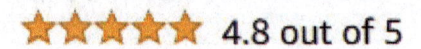

★★★★★ 4.8 out of 5

399 global ratings

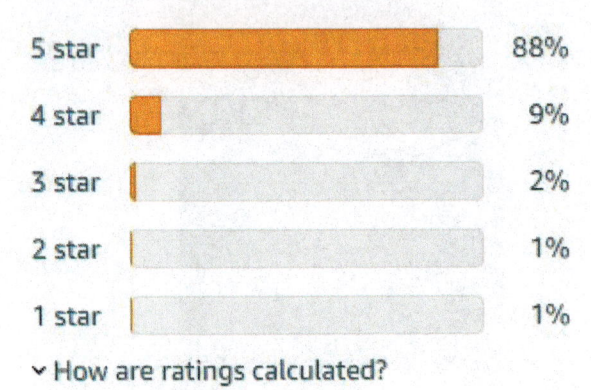

5 star	██████████	88%
4 star	█	9%
3 star	▎	2%
2 star	▏	1%
1 star	▏	1%

▾ How are ratings calculated?

Review this product

Share your thoughts with other customers

[Write a customer review]

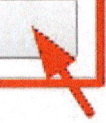

Hello, Dear Reader!

You've reached the end of the book — congratulations!

Thank you for reading Arthritis Action Guide & Cookbook, Easy and Tasty Recipes with Pictures

I hope you enjoyed it!

If so, would you please take 30 seconds to leave a quick review on Amazon?

Plus, it helps me produce more books like this in the future!

Here's where to go to leave a review now:

https://www.amazon.com/review/create-review/?ie=UTF8&channel=glance-detail&asin=B0C2H4DR83

Printed in Great Britain
by Amazon